Laughter for the Health of It

Kelley T. Woods

Dave Berman

Foreword by Madan Kataria, MD

Good Words

"When I was nineteen someone gave me a cassette that changed my life. The tape was of a group lead by one of my favorite authors, Robert Anton Wilson, and the only thing on it was laughter. There were raucous guffaws, high pitched chuckles, belly laughs, subdued giggles, and snorts. It was wave after wave, a tapestry of laugh as soundscape. It was impossible not to join in. I found it irresistible and listened at least twice a day. I found myself playing it for others and we would sit around my east village apartment laughing. It was contagious. I rode the wave of laughter right out of my depressive episode and used that tape as a magic wand whenever I had a friend in need.

Kelley Woods and Dave Berman share insights into why that daily laughter was so healing for me. They put together a collection of techniques and processes to share with groups, clients, family and friends that cultivate laughter as medicine. The idea of "unconditional laughter" is something we would all benefit by exploring."

- Melissa Tiers, author of *Integrative Hypnosis: A Comprehensive Course in Change, The Anti-Anxiety Toolkit: Rapid Techniques to Rewire the Brain* and *Keeping the Brain in Mind: Practical Neuroscience for Coaches, Therapists and Hypnosis Practitioners.*

"Full Disclosure: Dave Berman was my room-mate at the HypnoThoughts Live convention about a year before this writing. He arrived at around three in the morning, and my

alarm went off at six that morning. Now, when I hear an alarm go off--even my own--I tend to be puzzled by the sound and then annoyed or even enraged at the thought of waking up. However, that morning, about the time that I figured out the obnoxious music was indeed my alarm, I heard another sound that confused me even more. I slowly realized it was Dave, laughing uproariously from the other hotel bed.

Once I was coherent enough to speak, I asked him what was so funny about my alarm, and he replied that years of Laughter Yoga had rewired his brain so that he now laughs spontaneously at frustration. Being in the business of applied neuroplasticity, I was intrigued.

When attending Dave's class at that convention, I found myself laughing spontaneously and indeed uncontrollably after just a few of the exercises he describes in this book; I also felt amazingly blissful. I was hooked.

Since that time, I've become a Certified Laughter Yoga Leader myself. The recovering addicts at the center where I teach Anger Management enjoy Laughter Yoga as a valuable tool for emotional regulation. I combine laughter with conventional techniques for my hypnosis clients. And I've learned to laugh at my own frustrations, making me happier, calmer, and more positive.

So now, a year later, this book by Woods and Berman has expanded my thinking about laughter as a therapeutic tool, providing new techniques and insights. I wish I'd had it a year ago, because I can see it's a great introduction to the power of laughter."

- James Hazlerig, MA, CHP, Certified Yoga Laughter Teacher, Harmony Hypnosis, www.hypnosisaustin.com

"From the moment I started reading I was sucked in. Over 40 years ago in my early days of clinical training, I vividly remember observing Virginia Satir working with a family. In an intense moment of emotional upset, she cracked a joke with the Dad and got the whole family laughing. She used laughter to change the state so that they could move from right and wrong to a place where they could listen and hear.

After the family had left, we asked her about her use of humor and she was so emphatic about the importance of humor as a therapeutic tool to move people to wellness. Laughter for the Health of It *is filled with tools and resources to facilitate our clients to gain control over their mood and physical states. I highly recommend* Laughter for the Health of It *and believe that it should be required reading for all health and wellness professionals."*

- Roger Moore, CHt, www.HypnosisHealthInfo.com

"Dave Berman and Kelley T. Woods strike a funny bone with Laughter for the Health of It. *The information in this dynamic, easy to read book is life-changing, and will have you adding more laughter to your life with each turn of the page. You will learn how truly beneficial this positive resource state is to your health and well being, and that laughter really IS the best medicine.*

They also give practical tips for clinical hypnotherapists to incorporate laughter into their hypnosis change-work as a powerful and dynamic tool. This book is a gem!"

- Stephanie C. Conkle, BA, CCH, NLP, Clear Life Results Hypnotherapy, www.clearliferesults.com

Foreword

I am so happy to have been asked to be a part of this book, because helping people improve wellbeing through the power of laughter is something I have been dedicated to for a long time. I was raised in a rural environment that embraced spontaneous laughter as a way of life and it was not until I moved to the city that I noticed not everyone shared that gift.

Later, through my practice as a cardiologist, I began to be interested in the healing properties of laughter. I was disillusioned with the limitations of pharmaceutical interventions and some aspects of modern medicine in general so I looked toward the natural healing abilities that everyone possesses.

In this way, I started the Laughter Yoga movement, which has grown to a size that amazes me. My hope is to have these wonderful exercises integrated into schools, retirement homes and even prisons.

So, it was with joy that I heard about Dave Berman and Kelley Woods' project, helping to spread the good word about laughter therapy. In this book, they not only talk about the history of laughter therapy, they also show the health benefits of laughter come from the same mind/body mechanism used in their hypnosis work for so many physical and emotional issues. They also make it practical by providing some great ways for integrating laughter into your daily life.

I hope that readers will embrace the ideas contained in this book and join our wonderful community of people who laugh just for the health of it!

Dr. Madan Kataria

Founder of Laughter Yoga Movement

Table of Contents

Introduction

We're so glad that you are reading this book. We love it when we can touch just one more person, like you. The information and ideas contained in this book will help improve not only your life, but the lives of people *you* touch, because that's how healing works. We are all constantly influencing one another - in person or remotely, intentionally or not - and it is our hope that you will not only learn and apply, but also share the fun and easy laughter-for-healing exercises that are presented here.

As hypnosis practitioners, we've known for quite some time the many benefits of allowing ourselves to smile and laugh. In fact, Dave regularly conducts trainings for other hypnosis professionals so that they might experience it for themselves and learn new ways to encourage clients to laugh for healing.

Kelley incorporates "laughter for the health of it" into her hypnosis work automatically, guiding clients to exercise their laugh track as one of the foundational approaches for feeling better because *people who feel better, heal better.*

A personal story:

> Dave had an odd experience in the fall of 2013 that turned out to be like fertilizer, catalyzing the growth of seeds already germinating in his mind about the connections between laughter and hypnosis...

> While walking down the street, Dave felt something smash into his leg. This caused him to pause in mid step, standing still like a statue. In that instant, the

first thought to cross his mind was that the impact reminded him of being hit with a snowball during childhood. He immediately realized there was no snow in Arcata, CA.

Following that, several hypnosis concepts occurred to him virtually simultaneously:

1. Dave's mind had sought a familiar frame of reference to account for an unexpected experience. Hypnotists call this a transderivational search.

2. This search, combined with the physical jolt that prompted it, served as what hypnotists call a "shock induction," a surprising experience that immediately prompts entrance into hypnosis.

3. The frozen stance caused by the instant entry to hypnosis was an example of full body catalepsy, a common phenomenon typically elicited by hypnotists in smaller ways as evidence to convince a person they are in hypnosis (for example, suggesting a hand can't be lifted because it is stuck to a leg or chair, or that eyelids have become so heavy they will no longer open).

All of the above crossed Dave's mind in a span of perhaps two or three seconds, at which point he started laughing with awareness of those thoughts, and a reflexive reach down to the point of impact on his leg. The cold slime on his finger tips further confused matters for another second or two until Dave noticed the shell fragments on the ground and realized he'd been hit with an egg.

He looked up at the car that had passed him and was now a half block away, still hearing young guys hooting and hollering out the window. Now in full roaring laughter, Dave's next thought was that somebody in that vehicle has incredible aim! From there, what felt like a profound insight arrived:

This was essentially an assault that Dave escaped unharmed - a drive-by egging. Rather than being remembered as traumatic, Dave was already laughing about it because his regular dedication and practice of laughter had trained his brain to respond this way.

The experience became a turning point for Dave, solidifying his thinking about the connections between laughter and hypnosis, and setting him on course to start speaking publicly about how he was already combining the two in his professional work.

As research for writing this book, Dave finally got around to reading another book he had previously heard about many times in relation to his laughter practice. Published in 1979, *Anatomy of An Illness* is the autobiography of journalist Norman Cousins that details his recovery from ankylosing spondylitis, a painful and debilitating deterioration of connective tissue in the spine. The primary remedies Cousins used were megadoses of vitamin C and laughter. His book included a Foreword by microbiologist and Pulitzer Prize winning author Rene Dubos, who wrote on page 18:

"The body's defense against infection depends in large part on the mechanisms of humoral and cellular immunity, but these mechanisms themselves are influenced by the mental state--as demonstrated by the effect of hypnosis on the Mantoux test. This test consists in the intradermal injection of tuberculin, an extract of tubercle bacilli. It is used to evaluate the likely response of the body to tuberculosis infection. A famous English immunologist has recently established, however, that hypnotic suggestion can obliterate the vascular manifestations of the Mantoux test--as neat a proof as one could wish of the influence that the mind exerts over the body. The tuberculin Mantoux reaction pertains to the kind of body response that immunologists designate 'cell-mediated immunity.' Since this form of immune response plays an essential role in resistance to important infectious diseases such as tuberculosis, and probably also in resistance to cancer, there is good reason to believe that the patient's state of mind can affect the course of all pathological processes that involve immunological reactions."

We consider it encouraging validation to find others suggesting a connection between the mechanisms by which laughter and hypnosis alter physiology. As you'll soon see, this is a central premise to this book.

One of the most powerful benefits of using hypnotic principles in life is an increase in Emotional Intelligence – the ability to sense and understand not only one's own emotions, but also those of other people and even animals. Additionally, being able to respond appropriately to these inner senses affords us autonomy over reactions, behavior and overall mindset.

Those of us who practice mindful hypnosis regularly find that we live with a certain attunement of attention that is not only manageable, but controllable. We have keen awareness that self control is available only through power of choice and automatically seek out options that best suit a situation, no matter how challenging. You might also think of this as being able to "change the channel" when it comes to how you are experiencing life!

Here's another personal story:

> A few years back, as Kelley waited for a client in her hypnosis office, a neighbor came running in, shouting that someone had not only crashed into her parked car, they had left the scene (but he got the license plate number). She stood up, went outside to inspect the damage, called the police who arrived promptly and provided the officer with the necessary information.

> This took about 15 minutes, following which Kelley returned to her office to prepare for a client who was due to arrive shortly. At this point, it suddenly occurred to her that at no time during this experience had she been feeling any stress. No worry, no anxiety, no resentment or anger. She had automatically moved into a state that allowed her to take care of business.

> Even better, Kelley was now in the best state of being to work with her client, who needed her to be out of her own head. It was an epiphany to realize that, after often *trying* to control her emotional reactions (and her physical ones, because the body is always responding to our thoughts and feelings) Kelley had now experienced a helpful automatic response. This

was a response that allowed her to move clearly and calmly through the required tasks without leaving any lingering negative residue!

This experience demonstrated to Kelley that she had been successful in raising not only Emotional Intelligence, but what she has coined as Hypnotic Intelligence (HI). Since then, she thinks about HI often, especially when she notices herself using it (although it's mostly beneath conscious radar and what she notices more are the results of its use) or when working with clients who are lacking in this ability and need her help.

Readers who are familiar with meditative and mindfulness practice recognize what we are referring to here. Staying out of stuck states that are anchored in the past or suspended into the future and instead being *in the moment* allows us to embrace life in a more pleasant and effective manner. The practice of laughter yoga and mindfulness are wonderful tools to help retrain the mind and body to be more present. Hypnosis offers a wide variety of tools that are customizable for the individual, incorporating visual imagery and indeed, all of the senses, along with the creative imagination.

When we guide ourselves (or a client) to imagine a different way to respond to life, we are laying down blueprints for using choice to achieve control. Creating new neural pathways takes advantage of neuroplasticity to expand the selection of choices and eliciting feelings of relaxation, comfort, or excitement triggers physiological responses in the body that takes advantage of bioplasticity (a newer term we'll discuss further on page 39).

This all means that, whether we are engaging in intentional mindful hypnosis or using unconditional laughter (laughing by choice without humor to prompt us), channels are opened for healing and improvement on many levels.

And as a person responds positively with increased comfort, improved sleep, behavioral control, etc., their Hypnotic Intelligence also responds and grows. They gain a deeper awareness of the power of their mind to affect all areas of their life experience. Once that veil is lifted, everything changes. Perhaps that is also why we consider ourselves to be *de*-hypnotists; waking people up to the incredible abilities they possess!

We designed this book for use by anyone. So, whether you are an individual looking for innovative and practical approaches to improve your health and life experience or you are a health and wellness practitioner with a passion to help others, please enjoy incorporating more laughter into your daily regimen.

"Always laugh when you can. It is cheap medicine."

~ Lord Byron

Chapter One   History of Laughter Therapy

Throughout this book where we talk about laughter, we're really discussing unconditional laughter - laughter without jokes or any other stimuli. The idea of using unconditional laughter as a method of gentle aerobic exercise, and as a means of supporting physical and mental health, is now commonly associated with an activity called laughter yoga.

The history of laughter yoga began in March 1995 with a medical doctor named Madan Kataria in Mumbai, India. The story of the origin of what is now a global health craze has been told many times. This telling offers an uncommon twist, placing the story in the context of hypnosis and setting the stage for the rest of this book.

As the story goes, Dr. Kataria was testing the premise that laughter is the best medicine. He gathered together a small group of people in a park where they told jokes and laughed.

They did this each day for a short while and found that after a little bit of time the jokes wore thin, getting rude and nasty and raunchy. People weren't enjoying it quite as much. Even though the group had grown in numbers at first, participation began to decline.

Not to be defeated, Dr. Kataria asked everyone to give him one more chance to make this work.

He then did a little bit of research about what happens to the body physiologically when laughing. What he found was that the body and the brain work together to produce the same effects whether laughter is conditional (inspired by something funny) or unconditional - meaning laughter consciously initiated for the purpose of feeling good and improving health.

This is very similar to what hypnotists have long understood: the body can't tell the difference between what is real and what is vividly imagined. The most current brain scanning technology supports this premise.

For example, when a person is in an fMRI machine (functional magnetic resonance imaging), parts of their brain will register similar activity whether they are exposed to an actual stimulus or it is hypnotically suggested that they imagine that stimulus.

Similarly, with laughter, whether laughing at a joke or laughing unconditionally the brain produces what we call "happy hormones." These are dopamine, oxytocin, serotonin, and endorphins. There is also a drop in production of the stress hormone cortisol.

In a later chapter we will explore in greater detail the ramifications of these particular biological changes. For now, note that the similarity between the premise in hypnosis and in laughter yoga is the inspiration for this book.

So Dr. Kataria discovered through his research that even laughter that *seemed to be* for no reason would in fact reliably produce physiological changes known to have many health benefits. He went back to the group in the park and together they made funny faces and sounds simulating laughter. The laughter quickly became real and contagious.

Dr. Kataria recognized the role of the diaphragm in laughter and realized laughing can be a cardio workout all on its own.

His wife is a traditional yoga instructor, which of course involves great emphasis on breathing. Thus, as the practice of unconditional laughter grew, it included more focus on the breath and took on the name laughter yoga, even though it does not involve the same kinds of stretching and posing.

Over time, different pretexts and games were created to inspire doing different types of laughs. We might laugh like Santa Claus or a dog or pretend to be a sprinkler watering the lawn. The variations are endless and in fact are constantly being augmented with new games or "laughter exercises."

From that park in Mumbai, similar "laughter clubs" began springing up all around the world. Now 20 years later Dr. Kataria estimates there are more than 10,000 laughter clubs in over 100 countries. That qualifies as a health craze!

Note: Be sure to read the final chapter in this book that includes a personal interview with the incredible Dr. Kataria!

Your co-author (Dave) attended his first laughter yoga session in February 2009. It was a seated class for older adults at a senior center in Carlsbad, CA. Class was led that day by a couple named Gaga and Khevin Barnes. Afterward, Dave did a video interview with the instructors in which they mentioned their pioneering work leading laughter sessions multiple times each day for people around the world who call in to laugh together by telephone.

That party line is still used today. Find the number in the resources section of this book or get it from Dave's video here:

https://youtu.be/GxtpeN8emDE

More recently, a similar set of daily international laughter calls began happening on Skype. Those details are also in the Resources section of this book.

Meanwhile, in the years since attending that first class in Carlsbad, Dave became a devoted regular laughter yoga practitioner. In 2012, he became a certified laughter yoga leader and now combines the principles and techniques of unconditional laughter with hypnosis for his private hypnotherapy and coaching clients, as well as when leading group laughter programs.

The logical next step was presenting these beneficial strategies to other hypnotists and coaches, which he started doing at the HypnoThoughts Live conference in 2014. That's where Kelley Woods took notice and the idea for this book emerged.

Dr. Robert Provine, a neuroscientist and Professor of Psychology at the University of Maryland and author of *Laughter: A Scientific Investigation,* has spent decades researching *gelotology* (the study of laughter and its effects on our psychology and physiology). Provine's work suggests that laughter is a form of communication and is part of universal human vocabulary. He posits that the level of ability to laugh is probably genetic but we'd like to add that laughter exercises can raise that ability, taking advantage of epigenetics – the ability to alter DNA!

Chapter Two   Making the Case

Health and Well Being Benefits of Laughter

One of our favorite aspects of using laughter therapy is that it doesn't require a person to engage in "positive thinking". Now this may sound contrary to healing, but it's important to know that in many cases of chronic illness, such as depression or pain experiences, being exhorted to "think happy thoughts" or repeat positive affirmations can be counter-productive and actually *increase* a person's suffering. This is because the learned helplessness - hopelessness cycle has taught them that they cannot maintain the happy mood and the suffering becomes even further entrenched.

A study conducted by psychologist Joanne V. Wood at the University of Waterloo revealed that when people with low self esteem were told to repeat self-affirming, positive phrases they actually felt worse about themselves following the exercise. It is suspected that they automatically countered the affirmations with contradictory, negative thoughts that further lowered self esteem.

Merely engaging in laughter exercises bypasses the need to "think" your way into a more positive state. In fact, being stuck in anxiety-causing thought patterns is a problem that many people have, so getting out of your head and giving yourself permission to laugh out loud at nothing is incredibly freeing!

Dr. Joel Goodman, at the 2014 World Laughter Summit, shared something that one of his patients who participated in a laughter program created: L A U G H T E R is an acronym for:

Love And Understanding Give Hope
Toward Emotional Recovery

Using the Power of Choice

Laughter loves company and by choosing to utilize laughter as a positive resource, people gain control over mood and physical states. You might enjoy this Native American story that further demonstrates the power of choice:

An elderly Cherokee Medicine Man was speaking to his grandchildren. He said to them,

"A fight is going on inside everyone who has a health challenge. It is a terrible fight and it is between two wolves."

"One wolf promotes pain and disease--he feeds on fear, anger, envy, sorrow, regret, self-pity, guilt, and resentment."

"The other wolf promotes healing and well-being--he feeds on laughter, joy, peace, love, hope, serenity and faith."

The grandchildren thought about this story for a minute and then one child asked his grandfather, *"Which wolf will win?"*

The old Cherokee simply replied, *"The one they feed."*

Imagine that engaging in laughter therapy is feeding the right wolf in you!

Here are some of the many other positive benefits of laughing:

As we understand more and more the crucial role that hormones play in health and happiness, it becomes relevant that laughing increases the production of endorphins, natural opiates that make us feel good, while decreasing cortisol, the stress hormone that plays a role in appetite regulation.

Laughter stimulates the creative part of our brain, helping with problem solving. It also, according to the Journal of The American Medicine Association, or *JAMA,* increases *catecholamines*, which boost mental alertness, memory and "interpersonal responsiveness."

Many people who experience pain notice that laughter eases their suffering for many reasons (we'll explain why in Chapter Eight).

Engaging in regular laughing improves the immune system in several ways:

- It's a de-stressor. Stress contributes to immune depression.
- Laughing actually increases the body's T-cell presence.
- It increases lymphocyte blastogenesis, which improves immune function.
- Laughing is much like yoga in that it provides an internal massage. The physical activity of laughing massages the heart, lungs, diaphragm, abdomen and liver.

- It also strengthens core muscles, which are vital to overall body health and vitality. Additionally, laughter exercises can be targeted to specific areas of the body for strengthening, such as the pelvic wall for addressing incontinence, (see Chapter Nine).

Another physical benefit of laughter is that it is good cardio exercise; reportedly, 100 laughs equal a 15-30 minute workout! In addition to an improvement in blood oxygen levels, with regular laughter practice, blood vessels become more adept at expansion, which is an indicator for reduced risk of heart attack. People who laugh habitually experience up to 40% less chance of having a heart attack!

In fact, Michael Miller and his research team at the University of Maryland Medical Center have studied the effects of laughter on people by using ultrasound measurement of artery blood flow and dilation. Using clips from movies with themes of comedy and war, the scans showed how a laughter response created a 22% increase in blood flow compared to a 35% reduction, due to artery wall constriction, following viewing of the stressful movie scenes.

This research suggests that laughter may help keep arteries healthy, reducing the risk of cardiovascular disease and it certainly influences the mental stress that is known to harm the artery lining.

Additionally, laughter can improve lung capacity as a person learns to breathe in an improved manner. It can also help clear mucus plugs, aiding in respiratory problems such as emphysema or asthma.

Benefits for Diabetics:

Research conducted by Keiko Hayashi, Ph.D., R.N., at the University of Tsukuba involved a group of volunteers who have type 2 diabetes. After exposing the group, post-dinner on subsequent evenings, to a 40 minute performance the researchers measured blood sugar elevations. The first night involved listening to a boring lecture and the second consisted of enjoying a comedy show. They found that while the participants' blood sugar levels increased following the meal on both nights, there was a much smaller increase after the comedy show.

This research suggests that "chemical messengers made during laughter may help the body compensate for the disease". Interestingly, the same response was noted when the study involved patients without disease, giving the conclusion that laughter is good for everyone!

There is evidence that demonstrates how laughing is actually a good "anti-aging" mechanism; that it slows down the rate of cellular decay. Endorphin and human growth hormone production increase when one engages with laughter.

Laughter is even great for young ones – it increases melatonin, known as the "relaxing hormone," in breast milk.

During breast feeding, the brain also produces the "bonding hormone" oxytocin, contributing to the early (and enduring) sense of connection between mother and baby.

As mentioned earlier, laughter also stimulates oxytocin production. That means we develop feelings of fondness, connection and even attachment when we share a laugh. We tend to like the people with whom we laugh.

Hypnotherapists understand "liking" as one of the principles of influence identified by best-selling author Robert Cialdini, PhD. Get your clients laughing with you and change work becomes much easier. Teach your clients to laugh unconditionally and you can help them anchor access to an incredibly powerful and diverse resource with which we are all born. We'll discuss creating and collapsing anchors in Chapter Nine.

Note, too, that despite the lack of typical get-to-know-you conversation during laughter club sessions, it is common for friendships to emerge among frequent participants. This can be attributed to the bonding nature of the experience.

Put simply, laughing *feels* good. One reason is because another hormone that laughter stimulates is dopamine. This is the brain's reward system, associated with feelings of happiness and even the euphoria of a drug high.

Dopamine also creates a receptive learning state. Think about the best teachers you ever had. They likely included humor in their delivery. Our point is these benefits are available even without humor, just by laughing unconditionally.

An important disclaimer: your authors are not medical doctors. The scope of our work necessarily forbids us from prescribing medication or diagnosing people (whom we call clients, not patients). Likewise, we do not technically provide "treatments" or "cures."

That said, we often work collaboratively with licensed medical and mental health professionals as adjunct or complementary care providers. That requires us to be educated about many health conditions and conventional approaches to treatment.

One of the most common examples is the use of antidepressants for mood disorders. Some of these inhibit the reuptake of dopamine (or serotonin, another of the "happy hormones" stimulated by laughter).

Inhibiting reuptake means the dopamine or serotonin created remains available in the blood stream.

Again, we cannot provide medical advice and never recommend changing or stopping medications without consulting the doctor who prescribed them.

Yet it should be clear by now, through your own personal experience and scientific evidence, that laughter is a mood booster, whether it happens spontaneously or as a result of the intentional use of any of the fun and easy-to-do exercises contained in this book.

The following information from Dr. Kataria is provided to help you determine if engaging in laughter therapy is safe for you or your clients:

Laughter yoga is not a substitute for medical consultation for physical, mental and psychological illnesses, but is a powerful natural complementary form of healing. It is like any other aerobic exercise and may not be suitable for everyone as it involves some physical strain and a rise in intra-abdominal pressure.

Some people may have pre-existing medical conditions and one should take reasonable precaution before doing laughter exercises.

It is contraindicated for people suffering from:

- Any kind of hernia
- Heart disease with angina pain
- Persistent cough with breathlessness
- Uncontrolled high blood pressure
- Incontinence of urine*
- Epilepsy
- Advanced (bleeding) piles and hemorrhoids or any bleeding tendencies in any part of the body
- Severe backache
- Any acute symptoms of cough, cold and fever

People who have undergone major surgery should wait at least three months before doing laughter yoga. If in doubt first consult a medical professional for guidance. Anyone undergoing physician-prescribed therapy that experiences improvements through laughter should seek the advice of their doctor before reducing dosage or stopping treatment.

Those suffering from heart disease and high blood pressure but who are stable on medication and can take a brisk walk for 30 minutes without any symptoms can do laughter yoga with advice from medical specialists. People who have undergone bypass surgery can also do laughter yoga after their stress test is normal.

Pregnancy is also a relative contraindication. Women with previous history of miscarriages and also those who are in advanced stage of pregnancy should take medical advice from specialists before doing laughter exercises.

People suffering from minor and major psychiatric disorders can participate in a laughter session except those who are not in touch with reality e.g. schizophrenia, Hyper mania (manic part of bipolar depression).

Before any laughter yoga session it is important to make the following announcement: *"Laughter yoga is like any other aerobic exercise. Should you experience any discomfort, please discontinue and get medical advice."*

*Some of our clients have noticed that engaging in laughter therapy exercises have actually improved bladder control. See our approach ***No Pee-Pee Hee-Hee***, on page 99.

Hope is Realistic

As a co-founder of HOPE Coaching, an empowering mindful hypnosis team, Kelley has found that laughter therapy fits perfectly into a model of mind/body medicine.

HOPE Coaching embraces the idea that it's not so much the experiences and conditions in our life that controls our levels of happiness, comfort and satisfaction, it's how we *feel* about those things that makes an impact.

In the movie version of Anatomy of An Illness, Norman Cousins says Albert Schweitzer once told him, *"Illness never stayed with him long. He was too inhospitable a host. Each patient, he said, carries a doctor inside him. Physicians are at their best when they give the doctor who resides in each patient a chance to work."*

Later, Norman mentions that he asks his doctor why he's gone along with the bizarre treatment when he didn't believe in it. The doctor replies, *"Because you believed. Because nothing else was working. Because I love you and I'm willing to try anything reasonable or otherwise. But don't ask me to believe in something that has only the most superficial kind of research validity."*

There have been compelling studies in the area of placebo treatment that demonstrate that a *doctor's belief* about whether the treatment will work or not exerts a considerable influence on the outcome for the patient.

In fact, in the book version of *Anatomy of an Illness,* Cousins ties this all together on pages 63-64:

> "The placebo, then, is not so much a pill as a process. The process begins with the patient's confidence in the doctor and extends through to the full functioning of his own immunological and healing system. The process works not because of any magic in the tablet but because the human body is its own best apothecary and because the most successful prescriptions are those filled by the body itself.
>
> [snip]
>
> Attempts to treat most mental diseases as though they were completely free of physical causes and attempts to treat most bodily diseases as though the mind were in no way involved must be considered archaic in the light of new evidence about the way the human body functions.
>
> Placebos will not work under all circumstances. The chances of successful use are believed to be directly proportionate to the quality of a patient's relationship with a doctor. The doctor's attitude toward the patient; his ability to convince the patient that he is not being taken lightly; his success in gaining the full confidence of the patient - all these are vital factors not just in maximizing the usefulness of a placebo but in the treatment of illness in general. In the absence of

a strong relationship between doctor and patient, the use of placebos may have little point or prospect. In this sense, the doctor himself is the most powerful placebo of all."

As HOPE Coaches who incorporate laughter therapy into our practices, we emphasize that embracing the idea that Hope is Realistic is crucial to our clients' success. Creating expectation and belief that what we are doing is helping makes all the difference when it comes to guiding people to let go of hopelessness and helplessness!

"Playing and laughing together, especially when we play and laugh in public, because we choose to, just because, is a profound, and, oddly enough, political act. Political, because when we play or dance or just laugh in public, people think there's something wrong with us. It's rude, they think, childish, a disturbance of the peace. Normally, they'd be right. Except now. Now, the peace has been deeply disturbed – everywhere, globally. And what those grown-ups are doing, playing, dancing, laughing in public is not an act of childish discourtesy, but a declaration of freedom, a demonstration that we are not terrorized, that terror has not won, that we refuse to let fear, anger, guilt or resentment win and rule our lives."

~ Bernie DeKoven

Chapter Three Practical Tips

Frequency and Duration

Some people ask us how often they should use laughter exercises. Our answer is, "As often as you want!" While it's important to consider general fitness, along with any infirmities or injuries that may limit your ability to laugh for extended periods of time, it's usually safe to engage at least daily with laughter therapy.

"We don't laugh because we are happy, we are happy because we laugh!"

~ William James

In fact, research shows that it is more beneficial to take several opportunities during the day for brief bouts of mental and physical breaks, what we like to call "recesses," than it is to engage in an hour long meditation. Using laughter therapy even for just a few minutes reboots your mind and your body, moving you out of chronic stress states and into healing states that enhance your everyday life.

Here are some great times to engage in laughter therapy:

First thing in the morning, especially if you had a less than restorative night: Many people suffer from poor quality of sleep and a laughter exercise can be restorative. Even for those who sleep well, utilizing a favorite laughter recipe will set the tone for the day.

Before enjoying a meal: Imagine using laughter to release physical and mental distractions, allowing you to engage in mindful eating. Paying attention to your food helps you not only eat slower, it helps you feel more satisfied with less food, preventing over-eating.

During transitions such as your commute to work or school, when moving between chores or tasks, or between interactions with people: Use laughter therapy to leave unnecessary mental and physical burdens behind and move forward during your day and especially after work so that you can engage freely in your leisure time. How about, after you turn off your car ignition, just remaining there for a few minutes, laughing in your driveway or garage?

Any time you feel tension building within: No matter who you are, what the quality of your health or situation is, everyone takes on daily tension. Use laughter therapy to stay ahead of it, reducing stress and anxiety.

To unwind for the night: Imagine using laughter as a segue for sleep; starting with a robust laughter recipe and then moving into a more soothing, calming one and combining it with some gentle imagery will carry you off to La-La Land.

The Power of Your Breath

Many meditative practices, including traditional styles of yoga, emphasize focusing on breathing. Hypnotists also commonly instruct clients to notice each breath as part of the hypnotic induction process, turning attention away from external awareness and orienting it inward. If we're always breathing anyway, why is it so important to pay attention to this? When we observe our breathing, it keeps us present in the moment.

The mind has a natural tendency to get caught up in stories about the past or concerns about the future. Returning attention to the breath is a way to interrupt this common mental pattern without resisting those thoughts (which only fuels their persistence), trying to remember mantras or affirmations, or otherwise resorting to the "positive thinking" that can sometimes backfire as we explained in Chapter Two.

When you mindfully observe your breathing, blood pressure and heart rate will naturally decrease. In addition, the vagus nerve relaxes. The importance of this cannot be overstated. The vagus nerve accounts for what we often call a "gut reaction" or "gut instinct." These common terms simplify the scientific explanation of the enteric nervous system, also called the "gut brain." Here is an excerpt from "Hacking the Nervous System," published May 26, 2015* by Gaia Vince:

> *"The vagus nerve starts in the brainstem, just behind the ears.*
>
> *It travels down each side of the neck, across the chest and down through the abdomen. 'Vagus' is Latin for 'wandering' and indeed this bundle of nerve fibres roves through the body, networking the brain with the stomach and digestive tract, the lungs, heart, spleen, intestines, liver and kidneys, not to mention a range of other nerves that are involved in speech, eye contact, facial expressions and even your ability to tune in to other people's voices.*
>
> *It is made of thousands and thousands of fibres and 80 per cent of them are sensory, meaning that the vagus nerve reports back to your brain what is going*

on in your organs.

Operating far below the level of our conscious minds, the vagus nerve is vital for keeping our bodies healthy. It is an essential part of the parasympathetic nervous system, which is responsible for calming organs after the stressed 'fight-or-flight' adrenaline response to danger. Not all vagus nerves are the same, however: some people have stronger vagus activity, which means their bodies can relax faster after a stress."

* http://mosaicscience.com/story/hacking-nervous-system

By any definition, hypnosis works "below the level of our conscious minds." Even if you know nothing about hypnosis, consider for a moment how many ordinary activities you do without thinking about exactly how to do each component - walking, operating a vehicle, bringing food from the plate to your mouth, etc. It is only through practice that these processes become automatic and governed by the subconscious.

Should breathing be included on the list of automatic, subconscious acts? Of course. But when you don't think about your breath, other aspects of your physiology affect how you breathe and the result can be anxiety, high blood pressure or any of many other physical or mental issues. All of this adds up to make the case for getting regular cardiovascular exercise. There are many ways to do this but perhaps none as simple, fun, easy, and gentle as unconditional laughter.

Breathing Exercises from Laughter Yoga (credit to Jeffrey Briar, The Laughter Yoga Institute)

Breathe in very deeply. On the first repetition, breathe out quietly (extend effort to exhale as deeply as possible, emptying the lungs). On the later repetitions, laugh out loud in place of the exhalation.

1. *Up The Front* Start with hands down by the sides, fingertips towards the earth. On the inhale, raise arms high up above the head (palms face forward). Lower arms slowly on the exhale.

2. *Hastasana (or Tadasana Urdhva Hastasana) (Arms Stay Above Head)* First, bring arms up above the head, place palms together. Inhale and exhale while keeping the arms up.

3. *Reverse Prayer (or Butterfly Wings, aka "Montalbanasana")* Bring backs of fingers together in front of the chest (thumbs toward sky); then hands go up and behind the head, fingers pointing down towards the earth (behind the back). Stretch elbows wide apart; inhale and exhale (keeping arms in position).

4. *Arm Stretch (aka "Salutation to the Fun")* Interlace fingers below the waist, palms facing the belly. While inhaling, raise the arms up: palms to the face, then rotate the palms forward and up, ending with palms directed to the sky. Take a big stretch, continuing to inhale deeply --- "Hold it, hold it..." --- release the hands as you exhale, lowering the arms gradually down to the sides.

Additional breathing exercises:

Washing Machine - Stand with your feet shoulder width apart and your arms out at both sides, bent at the elbow with your hands beside your ears. Become the spin cycle of your washing machine, twisting gently from one side to the other so your hands alternate coming in front of your body. With each twist, forcefully exhale through your nose. Experiment with the speed, ranging from comfortably easy and slow to fast and challenging.

Pick a Flower - Reach down to the ground and pretend to pick up a flower. Take a deep whiff and exhale with a small chuckle. Share your flower with those around you and enjoy breathing in what they offer you. This is often used to slow the pace of a laughter yoga session after a more vigorous exercise.

Solo Laughing

While there are obvious social benefits of laughing with others, whether those are family members or friends, or as part of a laughter yoga club, there are folks who aren't comfortable laughing in this way. In our hypnosis practices, we have met many people who have lived in depressed, anxious or otherwise painful states and the idea of laughing is pretty foreign to them. They may even have forgotten how to laugh and the thought of laughing out loud in front of others is the last thing they want to do!

Kelley worked with a client who had such an aversion. This sweet lady, upon hearing of the benefits of laughter therapy, immediately stated, *"I could never do that!"* It was no surprise, since she had struggled with depression for quite some time and even confessed that she *wished* she could experience the joy and happiness that she saw in others.

She did agree to try some laughter exercises during the hypnosis session, so Kelley proceeded to engage her in a light trance, which reduced some of the inhibitions. Using the Giggle Factor exercise (see page 49) Kelley helped this client begin to chuckle freely, which lasted for several minutes. Upon returning to normal, waking awareness she was amazed at how easily she was able to laugh and, at how good it felt!

Being able to do this once created the belief and the momentum that this client needed and she began to practice laughter therapy on her own, lifting herself up out of a once depressive, hopeless existence.

TIP FOR HYPNOTISTS: When emerging a client from trance, imagine telling them that as you begin to count them back to full awareness they will find a giggle forming...increase that suggestion so that when they open their eyes, they are giggling, chuckling and even laughing seemingly for no reason, though of course those good feelings and health benefits are plenty of reason after all. Works like a charm!

Private laughter therapy is the perfect solution for people who are self-conscious or prefer to engage in self improvement on their own. As hypnosis practitioners, our primary role is to teach our clients how to raise their emotional intelligence and how to self-regulate not only thoughts and emotions, but physical responses, too.

When we are talking about improving emotional intelligence, the goal is to not only learn what our senses are signaling and how to respond effectively to them, but also to be aware of and able to understand other people's emotions. Becoming adept in this way positively affects communication on all levels.

We have found, also, that we share Dr. Kataria's view in that it is important to practice what we teach. He engages every morning for 30-40 minutes in Laughter Yoga and this is one of the ways that he creates the energy and motivation to achieve all that he is doing.

Self care is vital to any wellness provider and we recommend that practitioners reading this book develop their own regular laughter routine. Not only will you feel better, you may come up with some of your own recipes and, of course, you will be better able to help your clients understand the value of what you are sharing. Consider it another example of the same need present during the hypnotic induction to "go there first."

Whether you are using laughter yourself or teaching others, please understand that the lasting value is in the regular use of it. Daily laughter exercise is the secret component when it comes to creating permanent changes in the body and mind, so keep with it. Luckily, there is an unlimited number of recipes for laughter, like the many described in this book and even more contained right there, in your imagination!

Chapter Four   Laughter Recipes

There really is no right or wrong way to laugh. In fact, one of the joys of practicing laughter yoga is discovering just how many different ways there are to laugh!

When training as a Certified Laughter Leader, there are about 40 "foundational exercises" that all leaders are taught, including the breathing examples in the last chapter. We'll present some of those basics here, along with other common laughter exercises and some we've made up ourselves. Note that these recipes are not rules to be followed but rather descriptions of how we have come to enjoy being playful. Where possible, credit is given to the original creator of the exercise and where omitted it is assumed to be created either by Dr. Madan Kataria at the School of Laughter Yoga, Jeffrey Briar of the Laughter Yoga Institute, or considered a "traditional" exercise in the spirit of folk songs that have been passed down through the ages.

But first, there are two special chants used in laughter yoga that are not exercises, per se, but rather signal from the group leader that it is time to transition between exercises. As such, they are used multiple times in every laughter club session and have come to be recognized around the world as the most familiar defining sounds of laughter yoga.

Both of these transitions involve clapping. The leader typically instructs that the recommended way to clap during laughter yoga is with the palms together so all the fingers line up. This gives maximum stimulation to the acupressure points that activate the body's energy meridians.

The first chant is "Very Good, Very Good, YAY!" Usually the laughter leader will start the chant while the energy from an exercise is winding down, or the activity has reached its designated conclusion. Often participants will not get to join in on the chant right away so the leader typically does it twice. By the second time through, everyone in the group has switched their focus back to the leader and added their voice to the group chant. The hand clap occurs once for each "Very Good" and then arms go up in the air when shouting "YAY!" This chant invites the enthusiasm of a child opening birthday presents or playing with a puppy for the first time.

The second chant is "Ho Ho, HaHaHa." This chant is done to the rhythm of the cha-cha: 1-2, 1-2-3. Usually participants will hop, skip or at least walk around during this chant, allowing more eye contact and a reorganization of each person's placement within the circle (this is not applicable to seated classes with older adults, described in Chapter Six). The leader will signal when to end this chant either by ending with a single "Very Good, Very Good, YAY!" or simply giving an arms up "YAY!"

Value Based Exercises

Even though this book shows that we take the subject of laughter seriously, the exercises in this section help condition us to *take ourselves less seriously*, or interrupt patterns of responses to everyday situations often found stressful.

When introducing laughter exercises to hypnotherapy clients, the practitioner may seek to utilize these as if they represent a kinesthetic swish pattern. As our brilliant and hilarious colleague, Melissa Tiers, often says, a little discussion of neuroplasticity goes a long way. In this case, the value of the exercises can be enhanced by explaining that their practice will lead the brain to re-wire how it is programmed to react (remember the story of Dave being assaulted with an egg?).

Self - Point at yourself and laugh. Alternately, "selfie" laughter: hold your arm out as if taking a picture of yourself and ham it up for the camera.

Cry - Start with arms stretched above your head and pretend to cry as you bend at the waist and stretch toward your toes. As you straighten up your back, gradually bring your arms up over your head while increasing the exuberance of your laughter. Repeat. (Dave notes this reminds him of early childhood when his mother would be goofy when he cried, and as he started to laugh she would always say, *"Don't make me laugh when I wanna cry,"* which would always make him laugh more.)

Don't Laugh - Ever notice that the harder you try NOT to do something, the more a part of you resists. You can challenge yourself to *"Don't laugh!"* and see what happens!

Bummers - Mention unfortunate event while laughing as if it is hilarious (examples: I'm getting evicted; I just lost my job; my partner just broke up with me; etc.). These don't have to be true statements, but there is more value when they are.

No Money - Turn your empty pockets inside out, or pretend your wallet is empty, and laugh that you have no money.

Then discover you have a lottery ticket and celebrating winning the jackpot!

Credit Card Bill - Pretend you are holding a big credit card bill and point to all the expensive items as you show it to others and laugh.

Arguments - Walk around making big gestures and shouting at other people while using only Gibberish or made up phony language (Gibberish is the international language of laughter yoga!).

Naughty Naughty - Wave your index finger at people as if shaming them for doing something bad while making sounds like "tsk tsk," "naughty naughty," and "nah ah ah." Of course, do this while laughing.

Mirror - Pair up with another person and take turns mimicking each other as if one of you is looking in the mirror, making wild gestures, facial expressions and laughter sounds. Be sure to maintain eye contact as this helps trigger the brain's "mirror neurons" that contribute to the contagious nature of laughter.

This can also be a solo laughter practice, whether with a real or imaginary mirror. In fact, Dave's morning routine starts with a few minutes of laughter while looking in the mirror, tapping all over his body, and hopping around.

Red Light, Green Light - The laughter club leader will call out "green light" indicating it is time to move around pretending to drive while making low level laughter sounds like a car put-putting along. When the leader calls out "red light" everyone freezes and laughs with full enthusiasm and volume until the light goes green again.

Gum In Your Hair - Walk around grossed out and embarrassed to find gum in your hair while you and your friends use peanut butter to extract it. (*Courtesy Dave Berman*)

One of the things we've come to understand by exploring neuroplasticity, both via hypnosis and laughter, is that it is actually a subset of the larger category *bioplasticity* (a word apparently "proposed" by Lorimer Mosely, Ph.D. in 2014*, though at least one commenter notes "autopoiesis" is a pre-existing term for this concept).

The brain is not the only part of the body capable of adapting and making new connections. Think of learning an instrument, riding a bicycle, or the motions involved in various martial arts. When practiced, the coordination of physical movements involved in these activities and others becomes automatic.

Dr. Mosely points toward many other examples, including the growth of muscles in response to weight lifting, the change in pupil dilation based on available light, and the thickening of skin on the heel when regularly walking barefoot.

Given that the scope of benefits available via unconditional laughter includes improved circulation, enhanced immunity, higher pain tolerance, and more, we believe that bioplasticity is a more useful framework than neuroplasticity.

* http://www.bodyinmind.org/time-to-embrace-bioplasticity

Bioplasticity also seems to be what Rene Dubos was describing on pages 13-14 of his Foreword to *Anatomy of An Illness* by Norman Cousins:

> "Even under the most urbanized conditions we retain the genetic constitution of our Stone Age ancestors and therefore can never be completely adapted, biologically, to the environments in which we live. Wherever we are and whatever we do, as Cousins says, we cannot avoid being exposed to a multiplicity of physio-chemical and biological agents of disease. We survive only because we are endowed with biological and physiological mechanisms that enable us to respond adaptively to an immense diversity of challenges. This adaptive response may be so effective that most challenges do not result in disease. If disease occurs, the adaptive response commonly brings about spontaneous recovery without the need of medical intervention. Ancient physicians were so familiar with this natural power of the organism to control disease that they invented for it the beautiful expression *vis medicatrix naturae*, "the healing power of nature.""

The passage above continues by saying Cousins connected the idea of nature's healing powers to the idea of homeostasis. But Dubos suggests it is different: "Instead of being simply homeostatic, the response of the organism corresponds rather to a creative adaption that is achieved by a permanent change in the body or the mind."

So again we have the idea of improvement through plasticity, and the idea that such adaptivity is natural and innate. It is precisely because we know that we can count on the mind/body to do this that we are able to stimulate the process intentionally with how we choose to live - our "creative adaptations."

Types of Laughter

One of the traits of a person who is resilient in life is flexibility, so we encourage you to develop a wide range of laughs. Many of these exercises are ripe for improvisation and variety, which will help you discover the diversity of "laughter voices" you possess.

Animals - Move, gesture and make laughing sounds like a lion, monkey, duck, horse or any other animal. Dave created a variant called *Cross Breeds* using the movements of one animal and the sounds of another. For example, a dog that clucks like a chicken, or an elephant that moos like a cow.

Moods - The gestures, expressions and sounds we make vary greatly based on mood and energy. Explore what it's like to laugh when shy. Try nervous. Then embarrassed. Imitate a villain doing an evil laugh. Notice the delightful strain in the cheeks and jaw when laughing in slow motion. Imagine being at a religious service and having to hold in inappropriate laughter when you hear someone fart. Allow yourself to exuberantly laugh in silence. Throw your arms out wide and laugh heartily with total abandon.

Sprinkler - Begin with one arm in front of you, elbow bent at a right angle so the hand touches the opposite elbow. Extend the second arm straight out and move that hand in an arc a few inches at a time, simulating the sound of a lawn sprinkler (ch-ch-ch-ch). When the hand reaches the end of its range of motion, incrementally bring it back to its starting position "spraying" laughter along its path (huh-huh-huh-huh). Reverse arms and repeat. Then use both arms as sprayers. Finally, remove the nozzle and have a water fight with your friends.

Around the World - Many places have names that lend themselves to laughter sounds, especially those that end with vowels. Say each place, and then everyone around can repeat it with the extended laughter sounds. Examples: laughter yoga was invented in India-ah-ah-ah; in Finland, they laugh in Helsinki-he-he-he; Mexicans laugh in Baja-ha-ha-ha. Some names that don't end in vowels: Yuck-Yuck-Yucatan, Kandahar-dy-har-har, Cle-he-he-he-veland. (*Courtesy Dave Berman*)

Laughter Center - Point to your throat, then your heart, then your belly, then your funny bone, then any other parts of your body and for each one discover that each part of you laughs with a different voice.

Hot Sand - Imagine walking on the beach on a very sunny day, hopping, jumping and otherwise staying light on your feet because the hot sand is burning them.

Gotta Pee - When you gotta go, you gotta go, but sometimes the bathroom is occupied. Do the pee-pee dance and laugh while you wait your turn.

Laugh Identities

"The more you expect from life, the more your expectations will be fulfilled. By laughing, you do not use up your laughter, but increase your store of it. The more you love, the more you will be loved. The more you give, the more you will receive. Life proves that truth every hour, every day. And life continues to surprise."

~ Dean Koontz, Life Expectancy

Whether we are aware of it or not, other people and characters imprint upon us, influencing our thoughts and behaviors in profound ways. Perhaps you have friends or family members who have a special laugh you would like to emulate. If you need some role models, you can look to a world of entertainment filled with distinctive and memorable laughs. Here are ten fantastic examples of laughter styles you may want to embrace:

Classic 7-Up commercial > http://youtu.be/RhedZQOFSSE

Ernie from Sesame Street
> https://youtu.be/Uf8nPDGuvdM

Fran Drescher from The Nanny > https://youtu.be/-O29ZA24Jao

Roseanne > https://youtu.be/8HqJIfHpags

Ricky Gervais > https://youtu.be/jUh3Zm9807U

Adele > https://youtu.be/GTETb_crULs

Beavis and Butthead > https://youtu.be/m1agaZinJHg

Cartoon Characters > https://youtu.be/iPf3G1NQUfo

Arnold Horshack > https://youtu.be/SroYBkesPCw

Robin Williams as Mork > https://youtu.be/B5X3JI3LHlE

Let's take just a moment to discuss the exchange between Orson and Mork at the end of that brief clip:

Orson: "Stop acting like a child. You have to start calming down."

Mork: "Au contraire, Mon Grandiose. The dullest people on Earth are the ones that think they have to calm down and set a pattern for themselves as they grow older. And that pattern dictates what they should be and gives them very little freedom to be who they are."

On second thought, perhaps that quote speaks for itself.

In case ten isn't enough, here is a bonus laughter video featuring Dr. Madan Kataria:

https://youtu.be/QvAkyoA7l4U

Happy Feet Laughter

"Everybody laughs the same in every language because laughter is a universal connection."

~ Yakov Smirnoff

We learned this laughter exercise from our friend and colleague, Nathan Welch, an incredible therapist helping children and families in the U.K.

Nathan was watching a documentary about an indigenous tribe in Papa New Guinea and noticed that these people rated their success and status on their ability to be happy. The chief was the happiest man in the village, which is a pretty cool way to run a meritocracy, when you think about it!

Whenever they wanted to generate more happiness the tribal members got together and started to dance and jump and the more they did, the happier they became. Fascinating things, dancing and jumping, and Nath got to thinking how useful and easy this would be to incorporate with his clients.

Here is how to use feet and laughter to create happy states:

Have you ever wondered about times when your feet have just been *so* happy? It's easy to remember times of kicking leaves, splashing in puddles, jumping, running and dancing...all times when feet are having such a great time.

You might even consider which foot feels the happiest or maybe you want to start smaller, with a toe. Focus on how happy one toe feels and then let that feeling spread to the next toe, and the next. Wiggle your toes a bit, letting them

45

express those good sensations. Now, let that happiness move over to the other foot, too.

Have you noticed that your toes and your feet automatically want to start tapping and moving around? Go ahead and let that happen – invite the happiness to spread and become even bigger. Imagine what happens as those feel good energies move upward from your feet.

Now it's time, if you haven't already, to start giggling. When you are ready, turn the giggles into an audible laugh. Time your laughter with the wiggling and tapping of your feet and toes. If you are able, stand up and begin to hop, jump, or dance. Let loose! Laugh from the happy feet place and imagine spreading all of that joy outward, even as you feel wonderful inside.

You can use this Happy Feet Laughter technique to move away from things that are not helpful and healing and move toward things that *are* helpful and healing.

One of our clients used her Happy Feet to laugh her way out into her garden every morning. Previously, she had spent way too much time sitting on the couch, immobilized by chronic joint pain. Within minutes, she learned how to use the motion of her feet, combined with the comfort-inducing properties of laughter, to get moving.

You should see her now: she's a regular at the local dance hall!

Our thanks go to indigenous populations the world over who can teach many of us the true art of being happy and in the moment.

Access Positive Memories

"At the height of laughter, the universe is flung into a kaleidoscope of new possibilities."

~ Jean Houston

Giggle Fest! Do you remember, as a child, just starting to laugh with a sibling, a cousin or a friend or maybe even a parent and before you knew it, it became unstoppable? Laughter is contagious, just like yawning, and most of us have experienced those types of silly, meaningless and prolonged laughing fits that left us feeling joyfully exhausted.

Close your eyes and recall such a time. Even if you can't remember one, pretend that you do; your inner mind doesn't distinguish between real and fantasy, so just go with it!

Really get in touch with the experience now. Notice all of the details of how liberating it feels to really laugh out loud - to even roll on the ground and hold your belly as those laughs burst out of you. Then you hear someone else laughing just as wonderfully and it doubles your laugh! You may even gasp for air...pausing for a break...until even MORE giggles and laughs erupt.

It feels SO good! You feel SO great! You laugh at yourself laughing. You laugh at your friend or your sibling laughing. It's all just so ridiculously funny and you find it impossible to stop laughing. Ahhhh. Enjoy.

If you ever have difficulty consciously remembering a laughter memory, visit YouTube and search for videos of people laughing. Watch and listen while you let the laughter "contagion: infect you, proving you will always remember how to laugh at least subconsciously. Here is a link to a classic favorite called Bodhisattva in the Metro that shows this phenomenon in action:

https://youtu.be/iVekS_cOVfM

The Monkey Laugh

Have you ever made a monkey call? It's really fun and kind of freaks people out when you break out with a monkey imitation in the middle of the grocery store...Kelley has been known to do this, to the great embarrassment of her children. She also knows that this is a wonderful application of laughter therapy: start slow and low, then increase the frequency and speed of your monkey laugh.

It goes like this:

"Hoo, hoo, hoo...hoo, hoo, hoo...ha, ha, ha, ha, ha, ha, ha...ha-HA, ha-HA, ha-HA!"

Feel free to hang your arms down low and move in circles as you laugh. It feels wonderful! (Don't blame us if you have a sudden craving for bananas...)

Extra Credit: Challenge others to "monkey" your monkey laugh. You might even build a bit of a competition out of it, seeing who has the "best" monkey laugh of all!

Laugh about Nothing and Turn up the Giggle Factor

"Let the giggles fill your mouth because nothing tastes as sweet as laughter."

~ Richelle E. Goodrich

One of the most effective hypnotic visualization approaches for teaching a person how to self regulate, whether it is for physical sensations or emotions, is by using the control room metaphor. Here's how we do it:

Imagine that you are entering a very special room that is located deep within your mind. As you do, you notice that it is vast and the walls are lined with banks of softly flashing colored lights. It occurs to you that this is some kind of control room...and you are right: this is a control room in which not only your anatomy is measured and regulated, but so are your emotions, hopes and dreams.

For the purposes of this book, I want to direct your attention to the area where your emotional feelings are calibrated and controlled. Specifically, imagine the controls for your sense of humor and even your giggle factor. You may see the measurement as some form of digital readout, or perhaps there is a lever or a dial or even a color-coded device.

Whatever you see is just fine. You might notice at what level that control is currently set; perhaps it's rather neutral or, if you were just thinking of something funny, it may be indicating a heightened sense of humor. What do you think might happen if you turn it up a bit?

What do you think might happen if you turn it up a lot? If you are curious and open to it, go ahead and do that now.

As you do, notice how that giggle factor almost feels like it is being tickled. It's a fact that your body is instantly responding to whatever you are thinking and when you are thinking of just laughing for no reason...your body delightfully responds. Go ahead...turn it up even more and enjoy the sensation of chuckling...giggling...you can turn it up to such an intensity that you can even start to laugh out loud.

Notice how great that feels! It feels great to giggle and laugh and it especially feels great to know that you are the one making it happen. Now you have a new tool for turning up the laughter factor and it's as easy as just imagining that control or gauge and then dialing it up. You may find that you want to do it, more and more!

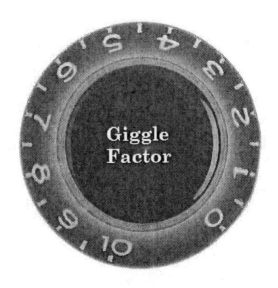

Do-Re-Mi-Ha - This is a fun one, especially if you can't carry a tune with a bucket! Use the classic scale song, substituting "Ha" for each note. Start slowly and then speed up with each rendition. Focus on your breath, making sure to take in a deep breath before starting up the scale and also before going back down again. (*Courtesy Kelley T. Woods*)

The classic lyrics:

Doe, a deer, a female deer

Ray, a drop of golden sun

Me, a name I call myself

Far, a long, long way to run

Sew, a needle pulling thread

La, a note to follow Sew

Tea, a drink with jam and bread

That will bring us back to Doe (oh-oh-oh)

(There are more song suggestions contained in the next section describing Group Laughter Activities).

Wicked Witch Cackle - Admit it, sometimes it's *so* fun to be bad. Channel the Wicked Witch of the East and notice what a good gut workout you get. You might even see some flying monkeys! (*Courtesy Kelley T. Woods*)

Yodel-a-Ha-Ha - No lederhosen required for this one, but you might find that you imagine yourself in the Alps, belting out a lovely laughing yodel. (*Courtesy Kelley T. Woods*)

Santa Claus - Feel the deep belly breaths as you laugh like Santa "HO-HO-HO."

Woodchopper - Clasp your hands together above your head with your fingers interlaced. Bring your arms down in three swift movements accompanying three forceful exhales of "HA."

Alooha - Similar to Woodchopper, but more gentle and drawn out. Reach both arms above your head and say "Aloooo..." and when you've held that stretch and breath long enough then slowly bring your arms down and exhale with a hearty "HA." Another version is to do a Hawaiian hula dance, swaying your hips and alternating waving arms on either side of your body while singing "Aloha-ha-ha-ha, Aloha-ha-ha-ha."

Shower Laughter - Pretend to take a shower and as you lather up let the imaginary bar of soap tickle you and release laughter bubbles.

Anti-Road Rage Laughter - While pretending to be stuck in traffic, or driving on a crowded roadway, discover what amusing laughter sounds your car horn can make (such as "A-OOO-GA").

Clean-and-Laugh - Move about pretending to do ordinary chores while laughing.

Chapter Five   Group Laughter Activities

"Laughter is the shortest distance between two people."

~ Victor Borge

A common denominator that we often find when working with clients who suffer from depression, anxiety, sleep disorder, pain and other chronic problems is a sense of isolation. We live in a world where one doesn't know their neighbors, where families are fractured and people are too busy to find the time to care for each other.

Many times, just having the opportunity to sit and enjoy a friendly conversation with us can make a world of difference to these clients. Unfortunately, we can't be there all the time for them, but we can inspire them to connect within their communities. Laughter yoga and other social laughing opportunities are a wonderful answer to the problems that isolation creates.

Even if there is not an organized laughter yoga club in your area, you may consider getting trained and starting one. Or, if you are a wellness practitioner, you may decide to incorporate laughter therapy into your regular group sessions or presentations. Laughing together is an excellent ice breaker and has been proven to increase social connections.

It is customary at the beginning of a laughter club session to tell the history of the founding of laughter yoga (though the hypnosis connection is typically omitted). This is usually accompanied by a very small number of rules:

1. No strain and no new pain. Laughter yoga is a gentle form of exercise suitable for all ages and fitness levels so participants are encouraged to modify activities to match their abilities and comfort levels. Some sessions are entirely seated while others involve frequent movement. It requires no special clothes, equipment or experience.

2. We laugh with each other, never at each other.

3. Generally there is very little talking, at least in regular words that invoke analytical left brain thinking. Laughter yoga invites the spirit of uninhibited childlike playfulness and creativity associated with the right hemisphere of the brain. When talking is encouraged, it is typically in the international language of laughter - Gibberish!

Laughter Greetings

One of the following is usually done near the beginning of each laughter club session:

Namaste - Mingle and greet each person with eye contact and palms together at your heart, bowing slightly and saying "Namaste" then giggling. *Celeste Greene* introduced a variant that keeps the bow but eliminates the word while everyone makes a face pretending to have no teeth.

Double Handshake - Mingle and greet each person by using both hands to simultaneously shake both of their hands, gently swinging your criss-crossed arms as you laugh together.

Electric Shock - Mingle and act as if you're about to shake each person's hand but as your fingers get close pretend to experience a static charge, jumping back with a shriek and a laugh.

High Five - Mingle and attempt to slap hands with each person but discover that you always miss and laugh about it.

Gunslinger - Mingle and approach each person with a suspicious look. As you get close to each other, reach in your imaginary holster and draw your hand with thumb up and index finger out, as if it were a gun. Point and shoot laughter at each other. (*Courtesy Kyle Wannigman, Arcata, California*)

The High Sign - The boys of *Our Gang* fame used the High Sign as their club's secret admittance gesture. Hold your hand, palm down, under your chin and wave your fingers. Emit a titillating giggle in time with the finger motion. We guarantee any witnesses to this will either immediately join you in laughing and high-signing back or they will run away! (*Courtesy Kelley T. Woods*)

FOLLOW THE LEADER EXERCISES

These are all designed as group exercises that allow each participant to spontaneously improvise any kind of laugh, which everyone else then imitates. These exercises are great for groups of up to 12-15 people, but may be too time consuming, repetitive or vigorous for larger groups.

Spin the Ha Ha - like the teenage party game Spin the Bottle, in the laughter version everyone sits in a circle. It starts with the leader spinning an imaginary bottle and then pointing to someone who then starts laughing. Everyone else imitates that laugh. Then the laugher "spins" and points to another person who laughs however they please, imitated by everyone else. Repeat until everyone has had a chance to inspire the group with their laughter. (*Courtesy Dave Berman*)

Conga Line - Form a single file with each person placing their hands on the shoulders of the person in front of them as everyone moves together repeating "ha-ha-ha-ha-ha-ha-HA, ha-ha-ha-ha-ha-ha-HA," kicking one leg out to the side on that final emphasized laughter note.

Canned laughter - Everyone in the circle holds an imaginary can. One person opens their can to discover what type of laughter comes out. Everyone imitates until the can is closed again. Repeat for each person in the circle. (*Courtesy Kathleen Krauss, Arcata, CA*)

Calcutta - This is traditionally a simple foundational exercise where hands are alternately pushed out in front of the body and then down while chanting "ho ho" and "ha ha." However, at the Humboldt Laughter Yoga Club where Dave practiced Laughter Yoga with Kathleen Krauss for three years, this exercise evolved into a more elaborate activity.

Instead of just the two simple sounds and gestures, any kind of movement and laughter sound may be offered while the rest of the group follows along. It often resembles a cheerleading squad on the sideline of a sports event. Each participant takes a turn leading.

Gradient - This is another simple foundational exercise that evolved in Kathleen Krauss's club in Arcata, CA. The original form has everyone start with a smile, then slight chuckle, then increasingly bigger laughter. Like the other follow the leader exercises, the expanded version of Gradient allows each person an opportunity to demonstrate a unique laugh to be copied by everyone else according to the calibration of volume and intensity demonstrated through some type of gesture. This could be an imaginary dial turned up and down, increased and decreased distance between two fingers or hands, crouching and standing back up, or any other depiction of less and more.

Silly Walk - Starting with a single file line, the first person walks in a silly way, such as with arms flapping, knee high marching, pretending to swim, etc. Of course some kind of laugh accompanies the silly walk and everyone in line imitates both the movement and sound until the lead person makes their way to the back of the line and the new head of the line sets a different example to follow.

Hand it to Laughter

Our hands are so special. Think about it, your hands are implicit in much that you do, helping you in unlimited ways. Why not recruit them into some laughter rituals? There are a bunch of handshake exercises and no limit to the ones we can invent...

The High Five - Take this popular congratulatory expression to another level when you add a resounding "Ha!" to meeting of hands.

Patty Cake Laughter - Remember this child's game? Here are some of the traditional lyrics:

Pat-a-cake, pat-a-cake baker's man

Bake me a cake as fast as you can

Mix it and stir it and bake it just right

Good from the first 'til the very last bite

"Laughter is important, not only because it makes us happy, it also has actual health benefits. And that's because laughter completely engages the body and releases the mind. It connects us to others, and that in itself has a healing effect."

~ Marlo Thomas

Echo Laughter - This is another great group laughter activity. One person is the primary laugh-styler and the others "echo". The echo versions are softer.

Gibberish Laughter - as noted earlier, Gibberish is the international language of laughter yoga because we want to avoid using our usual language processing and left brain thinking. Arguing in Gibberish is a great way for couples/family members to ease tension and for an individual to engage stubborn parts with an internal pattern interrupt. Gibberish can also be used in an imaginary cocktail party setting for pretend flirting or casual conversation.

One other common use is *Gibberish Punchlines*, where one person steps into the circle and "tells a joke" using only Gibberish. The inflections and gestures help the rest of the group know when the joke is over and it is time to laugh.

Sing and Laugh

Convert the lyrics of your favorite songs to laughter. There are no limits when it comes to butchering music for your own benefit!

In fact, on October 9, 2014, Dave Berman was leading a laughter yoga class at Moonlight Beach in San Diego when Giovanna Iaffaldano, during her first ever laughter yoga class, suggested they improvise a Doo-Wop song. The group split into sections, each choosing a laughter pattern to repeat in harmony, and all the sections sang their parts simultaneously as if producing the results of a multi-track recording.

Hokey Pokey - Just like when you were a kid, you put your left arm in, you take your left arm out, you put your left arm in and then you shake it all about. You do the Hokey Pokey and you turn yourself around. That's what it's all about. You can actually do the song and dance for various body parts or just replace the words to the song and sing it with core "HO" and "HA" laughter sounds.

Other good laughter songs:

Row, Row, Row Your Boat - Sing it with laughter sounds or the actual words, but definitely sing it in rounds. Another good song is *This Old Man*.

Take Me Out To The Ballgame - Another one that works with real lyrics or laughter sounds, this nostalgic song is especially popular for groups of older adults living in managed care facilities.

Ha Goes The Weasel - Use the "HA" sound while cranking your arm in a circle and gradually crouching down. As you get to the final "HA," reach your arms up and jump to "POP" the weasel (like a Jack-In-The-Box).

Mexican Ha Dance - Skip around linking arms with others as you sing "HA-HA-HA-HA-HA-HA-HA-HA-HA, HA-HA-HA-HA-HA-HA-HA-HA-HA, HA-HA-HA-HA-HA-HA-HA-HA-HA, HA-HA-HA-HA-HA-HA-HA-HA!" (that's three sets of 9 HAs followed by one set of 8). Get faster with each round.

Tequil-ha - This 1958 mostly instrumental Latin-rock #1 hit song by The Champs is known for its "dirty saxophone" part and the gravelly voice that periodically says "Tequila." It is has since been recorded by many other bands and has been widely referenced in pop culture over the years, perhaps most notably in the scene from the 1985 movie *Pee-wee's Big Adventure* in which Pee-wee Herman first angers a biker gang and then wins them over by dancing to this song. Its familiar rhythmic groove easily translates to laughter sounds and lends itself to doing the Pee-wee dance.

Ha-va Nagil-ha - Use the "HA" sound to the familiar tune based on the 100 year old Hebrew song popular at Jewish weddings, Bar and Bat Mitzvahs, and various sporting events around the world: "HA-HA, HA-HA-HA-HA-HA, HA-HA-HA-HA-HA, HA-HA-HA-HA."

By the way, here is the English translation of the real lyrics:

Let's rejoice, Let's rejoice, Let's rejoice and be happy

Let's sing, Let's sing, Let's sing and be happy

Awake, Awake, my brothers! Awake my brothers with a happy heart

Awake, my brothers, Awake, my brothers! With a happy heart

Orchestra - This brings us full circle to another foundational exercise in which one person conducts and the rest of the group becomes a human orchestra, with each individual acting out the motion of playing an instrument while it produces laughter sounds. Take turns being the conductor and feel free to change your instrument between songs.

Chapter Six   Laughter for Older Adults

"You don't stop laughing because you grow old.
You grow old because you stop laughing."

~ Michael Pritchard

The aging population in the West is growing at impressive rates, with the number of older adults estimated to reach nearly double 2012 figures by the year 2050!

"The United States is projected to age significantly over this period, with 20 percent of its population age 65 and over by 2030," said Jennifer Ortman, chief of the Census Bureau's Population Projections Branch.

As the Baby Boomers move into retirement age and beyond, we will be looking for more affordable solutions to the challenges they face.

Celeste Green is a Certified Laughter Yoga Teacher and the founder of Laughter Yoga Atlanta. She earned her Master's degree in Gerontology (the study of aging) at Georgia State University, in part by studying laughter among older adults in various community living centers.

The most common issues Celeste observes among older adults are memory loss, limitations on mobility, social isolation (feeling invisible), and a loss of autonomy, particularly after giving up living alone.

In residential facilities for older adults, Celeste says, *"Allowing them to choose to laugh, I believe, brings about this sense of autonomy...when older adults come into these laughter yoga classes, and choose to let go, something beautiful happens. They begin to gain a sense of control of their lives. But also, they begin to have a meaningful connection with people who are essentially strangers."*

Celeste says there are four key elements that contribute to a sense of well being and joy in older adults. These are:

1. singing

2. dancing

3. laughing

4. play

Group laughter activities go a long way to relieve that sense of isolation, uniting older people not only with each other, but with younger participants. Laughter is great common ground for people of any age and of any background, for that matter, and can lift participants up from depression and loneliness.

"Since laughter helps with bonding," notes Celeste, *"people come together, they laugh together, and really feel a sense of friendship. And I think that's what separates laughter yoga from a traditional exercise class or any kind of engagement activity, like bingo, for example."*

Laughter therapy eases feelings of fear and insecurity and builds self esteem. One might even think of laughter therapy as being the best form of social networking for this population!

Chronic health problems are quite common among older adults. Up to 80 percent of this age group experience one such issue and 50 percent have at least two. Clearly the "Golden Years" aren't always rich in good health and joy.

Cognitive declines limit many older adults from participating in interactive activities, but laughter exercises are suitable for people who suffer from dementia or Alzheimer's. Because of the simplicity of the laughter recipes, which do not rely on engaging in humor, they are easy to practice. In fact, research shows that people with these degenerative issues often find improvement in memory and other cognitive function.

Older adults who are less physically active, due to age-related infirmities or just a sedentary lifestyle, reap not only renewal of the mind but they also enjoy the fitness benefits of laughter therapy. Because the exercises are low impact, most people can participate in them.

In Celeste's original Master's thesis research she found a spike in mental health and also aerobic endurance and self efficacy for exercise. *"Of those scores,"* Celeste says, *"I was most excited about aerobic endurance because this program was done while seated. So just going through the motions really could mimic aerobic exercise for this population in terms of heart healthiness."*

Laughter therapy combines all of these vital elements within easy, fun, and dynamic exercises. We want to emphasize the FUN factor. Fun is what motivates people choosing to keep participating. Some older adults may find it easier to give themselves over to playing laughter "games" rather than "exercises," which they might have convinced themselves they're no longer capable of doing. Others may need to watch their peers a little first before releasing resistance to playing with the group.

Celeste also shared with us some things to keep in mind when working with older adults:

- Keep language simple and concise. People with cognitive decline may only be processing 1 in 4 words. You can slow your speech and actions down, also, but please avoid using what is known as "Elder Speak" – a condescending form of baby talk that people mistakenly use when communicating with older adults.

- Go physically to their level. If they are sitting or reclining, be sure to adjust your height for best communication and rapport.

- Manage your expectations. Just because a participant isn't making a lot of noise during the activity doesn't mean they aren't getting a lot out of it. Many people who merely chuckled later reported how good it made them feel.

- Define success on their terms, not yours. "Use value based exercises based on what participants find stressful. This could be lost glasses, or a lost mind," says Celeste.

- Invite participation but don't pressure people to join in. This is a fun activity but it's not for everyone, at least not at first! This is good advice for facilitating laughter with any age group.

- In our hypnotic work with older adults, it has been clear that long term memory banks are a wonderful realm for imaginative play. Laughter exercises prime and cultivate the imagination, so use imagery and references to all sensory systems, especially nostalgic music selections. "Rhythm and song are among the last things to go," says Celeste.

Some of the traditional children's songs from the previous sections work well with older adults. Another one is the Happy Birthday song. Remember, this can be sung with the actual words or just laughter sounds.

Here are some additional differences that come with doing laughter yoga specifically for older adults as compared to an open public laughter club.

- Participants are likely to all be seated and should not be expected to jump, skip, hop or run around. Activities should necessarily be lower impact both physically and aerobically.

- In addition to drawing upon nostalgia, the familiarity of recent laughter exercises can help older adults feel more comfortable so repeating games or songs is more appropriate.

- Their attention spans and commitment is often less so a shorter program may make more sense.

- Leading laughter yoga in an older adult residential center often includes the benefit of having paid staff members present who enjoy established relationships with the residents because they care for them every day. Involve the staff members in the laughter exercises. The residents may be more inclined to follow their lead than yours.

- Be sure there is water available for everyone.

- Don't get thrown off if one or more people sit in the circle without full participation. It is OK to gently encourage but do not single anyone out. Some may prefer just watching and enjoying the action!

- Likewise, don't take it personally or get upset if anyone leaves before the session is over.

- Model the behavior you want to see, but realize that your level of enthusiasm and exuberance may be intimidating or overbearing. Calibrate to your participants, and again rely upon any attendants to give you cues.

Note: While there may not be any laws about this, or guaranteed repercussions for ignoring this suggestion, we strongly recommend that you complete formal laughter yoga leader certification training prior to taking on a group laughter facilitation role, whether for older adults or any other demographic.

When you are properly trained, setting up opportunities to lead laughter groups for older adults may be best approached differently than for an open public group. Don't count on social media or flyers on community bulletin boards to attract people to a location you've chosen for them. Instead, be willing to go where they are.

Start by approaching activity directors across what Celeste calls "the continuum of care," ranging from independent living centers, assisted living, senior centers, and skilled nursing facilities. Be ready to provide some education, perhaps even offering a copy of this book, as not everyone is aware of laughter yoga and its many health benefits.

In such a setting, it is appropriate to accept payment for your services, though despite any other credentials you may have the compensation rate for laughter facilitation is likely to be on par with whatever is paid to leaders of others kinds of activities at the center. Note that being paid in this setting contrasts with leading open public laughter clubs where it is customary to volunteer (donations can be accepted, typically just to offset any costs if the space used must be rented).

Chapter Seven
Laughter for Children and Teens

It's easy to assume that children are natural laughers and there is even an urban myth that espouses how children laugh 400 times a day, compared to an adult's mere 15 times. While children do tend to be more in the moment and able to enjoy life as it comes, the truth is that levels of anxiety and depression in children are on the rise.

Research demonstrates a dramatic increase in the occurrence of depression and anxiety in children over the last fifty years. One recently released study, conducted by experts at San Diego State University, examined research that compared young people's sense of control and found that a higher level of anxiety and depression was correlated with a lower level of sense of control over external influences. In other words, the more children worried about things outside of their personal, intrinsic control, the more they suffered from mental distress.

Carol Dweck, in her popular book, *Mindset*, makes the point that children do not build self esteem and create success by being told how good, smart, able, etc., they are; instead, it is through experiential lessons that they become equipped with the confidence and skills required to thrive in life.

When working in the area of pediatric hypnosis, we recognize the value of empowering children with a sense of control. Teaching them to self-regulate not only emotionally, but physically, is one of the common goals with the hypnotic approach. And when it comes to teaching someone of any age something that you want them to learn, if you make it FUN, they will learn it easily. Laughing is fun!

Many modern children are really lacking in the area of play. With over-filled, adult-managed schedules, kids are on task from their early waking moments through a busy day, often engaged with activities until late at night. The loss of play and free time is taking a toll on young people, not to mention overall family well being.

Our friend and colleague, Michael Ellner, often mourns that too many people of all ages suffer from FDD – Fun Deficiency Disorder! Imagine using laughter techniques on a daily basis, to provide a fun and light-hearted approach to the *seriousity* of life. Incorporating some of our laughter exercises into your family's daily routine will not only help you help your child alleviate tension and stress, it will help them stay ahead of it.

This book is armed with recipes for laughter but, of course, you can also make up your own! Kids are filled with creativity and will quickly invent fun and crazy laughter exercises. When you engage children with finding solutions through play, amazing things happen.

Some families who really get into this start a Laughter Recipe File, decorating a recipe box or book and filling it with 3 x 5 index cards containing their laughter ideas. Randomly choosing the "Laugh of the Day" makes healthy laughter a regular part of your family's lifestyle.

TIP: Make laughing with older adults a part of your child's experience – these two age groups need each other for a variety of reasons! If you don't have any in your family, reach out into the community and find some.

There are unlimited opportunities for you to engage your children with laughter exercises:

- When waking them up in the morning
- Before enjoying a healthy meal
- During commutes to school or activities
- As a part of traditional Family Night
- Making laughter recipes a ritual for starting the weekend
- To complement household chores
- While in the bathtub
- Laughing away stress at the end of the day

Here are some childhood problems that can be addressed with laughter therapy. Please be sure to consider any of the possible contraindications we mentioned earlier in this book before proceeding.

Pain

Research has shown that distraction is a great pain reliever for children. Distract them with the silliness of laughing intentional and unconditional laughter and watch them get in touch with more comfortable sensations. Not only does laughter help reduce the emotional suffering that comes with pain and illness, it elicits physiological changes in the body that improve comfort levels.

Combining visual imagery, along with other senses, is easy to do with children. Children are mostly in nice little trance states and children in pain are particularly suggestible. Utilize those amazing creative minds with exercises that help them laugh the pain away.

TIP: It's not necessary to have children who are suffering exert themselves – even a gentle laugh will trigger relief.

Blow up the Pain Balloon - Tell the child to imagine a balloon is sitting on their shoulder or if they are lying down, on their belly. (What color is it?!) Show them how to breathe out as they laugh, inflating that balloon...making it grow larger and larger. It's filling up with all of that pain, all of that discomfort. Hey, as they change their laugh, the balloon starts to float up, up, toward the ceiling, maybe even up through the roof and into the sky.

What would they like to do with that pain-filled balloon? Shoot it to pieces? Let it fly up into the Milky Way?

Tip: Avoid asking the child how they feel now or worse, what their pain level is like. Just let them enjoy the residual feeling that came from having fun.

Be like a Noodle - We know that tension leads to pain, so helping a child relax physically will make all the difference when it comes to pain relief. We teach breathing exercises to children as young as 2 or 3; when it is framed as a fun game, they easily learn to use their breath to release the pain.

Combining easy, simple breathing techniques with soft laughter can be a good tactic for kids. You might ask them what a wet noodle feels like, looks like and laughs like. We guarantee, if you've never heard a wet noodle laugh, it's really something!

Float and Fly - One of our best hypnotic tricks involves dissociating from the physical body. Children love to let their body just stay down there, while they float around at the top of the room. If you've seen that great movie, *Charlie and the Chocolate Factory*, you may remember the scene where

Grandpa Joe and Charlie steal some Fizzy Lifting Drink and float. They get in a bit of trouble and finally are saved by burping their way back down. Imagine making a version of this for a child – wherein laughs elevate them out of their body. If necessary, encourage making burping, farting or other noises that will inevitably turn to laughter.

Anxiety and Fear - Did you know that monsters are allergic to laughter?! Well, at least the mean monsters are and that means that anytime a kid laughs, a monster runs away! Join your child in a laugh around the room to clear out any fears.

One of the reasons that people (kids are people, too) become fearful and anxious is that they are spending time worrying about what they are afraid might happen, rather than thinking about what they want to happen. The creative imagination is managed differently than conscious, rational thought and has the ability to *suspend disbelief*, making those fears come alive.

Laughter therapy provides the venue for re-scripting those fears and worries, instigating narratives and visions of silliness, strength, courage and survival that supercharge a child's resilience and personal confidence. Invite your child to tell you a story about a superhero or imaginary friend who overcomes a challenge. Such stories often lead young people to discover their own solutions, or identify what they need from their caregivers in order to feel safe.

Grief and Loss - Children don't usually know how to express their grief and because the emotions feel strange and uncomfortable to them, they often suppress them. Imagine helping your child discharge the sadness and pain of loss through the magic of laughter. You can help them model laughter – what did Grandpa sound like when he laughed? Can a dog laugh? You get the idea. Using our exercises appropriately can help keep the deceased's spirit alive when the house fills with laughter.

"I believe that imagination is stronger than knowledge. That myth is more potent than history. That dreams are more powerful than facts. That hope always triumphs over experience. That laughter is the only cure for grief. And I believe that love is stronger than death."

~ Robert Fulghum

Laughter for Physical Exercise Benefits

Jump Rope Laughter – Kids can jump rope (real or imaginary) for a certain number of laughs or for a specific amount of time. Other kids can participate, too, turning the rope and laughing along.

Rabbit Hop Laughs – Hop. and laugh. This one is for young knees!

Lava Laughter -Who hasn't played "Keep out of the hot lava"?! Add laughter to this exciting favorite. An added feature may be that he who falls in the lava has to come up with a new way to laugh in order to be rescued. Or, let the kids create their own rules - that's the best way, anyway.

Laughter for Sleep Preparation - Helping a kid wind

down for sleep is another way to use laughter exercises, believe it or not! You can use the "Be a Noodle" approach or, the Tap-n-Laugh recipe is great for kids. Sit on their bed and gently tap with them as they laugh softly. This helps discharge pent up tension and energy from the day, moving them into a relaxed state for sleep.

Trouble - Instead of sequestering an unruly child for an isolated time-out, how about engaging them in a laugh? Kids like props and using a 3-minute sand timer will intrigue them.

Family Laughing Games Night - The family that laughs together, sticks together. Use laughter games to help your family bond. You might think about having a special night once a week (or more!).

Commute Laugh - We mentioned earlier that taking advantage of daily commutes (or long road trips) are ideal places for laughter therapy. Leading your family in a laughter exercise will help everyone stay in the moment and more importantly, stay connected with each other.

TIP: When working with younger kids, under the age of 10 or so, limit the number of laughter exercises to no more than three. That's plenty to get them involved but won't overwhelm them.

Laughter for Teens

One of the most important things to know about teens is that they are often self-conscious about laughing out loud, especially in front of people they don't know and feel comfortable with. So, if you are instigating some laughter therapy in a group of teens, take into consideration the social dynamics. It may be preferable to break them into smaller groups to start with, keeping them age or gender specific.

It's also helpful to manage your own expectations of how they will engage in the laughter exercises. Just because an individual teen isn't particularly loud or demonstrative with a technique doesn't mean that they aren't getting anything out of it.

We have found when working with teens in our hypnosis practices that they are extremely interested in the science and in the art of how their minds and bodies work. When we create belief that a particular approach will help them self manage, gaining a higher degree of personal control, we usually capture their attention in a big way. So, presenting laughter therapy as a modality for self-improvement and independence is a motivating angle when it comes to getting teens on board.

Of course, many teens are still very childlike, thank goodness, so playing up the fun factor is the ultimate hook to capturing their imagination and participation. This means that as an adult, you need to unleash your own inner child and get into the laughter as easily as possible.

You will also gain a better chance of getting young people to engage with you in laughter therapy if you have some familiarity with their vernacular, their pop culture, icons, etc. Do a bit of research if you don't have teens at home to bring yourself up to date on current trends and then adjust the laughter recipes accordingly.

If you are laughing with your own teens, do be sure to incorporate some of your own family history and inside traditions and rituals.

Chapter Eight

Laughter for Reducing the Suffering of Pain

"Laughter is the tonic, the relief, the surcease for pain."

~ Charlie Chaplin

Hypnosis has many answers for people who have chronic pain. We know that all pain actually occurs in the brain (so when a doctor says, *"It's all in your head,"* well, it really is!) What a person experiences isn't the sensation in a particular afflicted area, it's their perception of it and how it impacts their life. That's why, often, an injured person may not even feel pain until they realize or see that they are hurt. It's also why mindset can play a big role in the level of suffering from chronic pain. Along with improving mental and emotional states, hypnotic techniques help people actually turn down or otherwise manipulate that pain signal.

Sometimes, even when an injury has healed, the nervous system can get entrained with the pain signal and keep sending that message to the brain. This unexplained pain can really wreak havoc with a person's sanity!

A Case Study from Kelley:

Joe came to see her seeking relief from his suffering of chronic pain due to Crohn's Disease and related osteoarthritis. He had a history of prescription medication abuse and was also a recovering alcoholic. Some of his depression was due to guilt that he had caused his family due to his addictions. His wife had passed away from cancer several years prior and he was still struggling with grief.

Joe had tried everything to alleviate his suffering, with little success. While he used a limited amount of pain medications, especially when damp weather exacerbated his symptoms, he was afraid of getting sucked back into abusing them and was open to other approaches. He arrived in Kelley's office in an obvious state of hopelessness. Her job was to install not only some hope, but also belief, that together they could find him some relief.

A quiet spoken, tall and solemn man, Joe lived alone and was frustrated that he wasn't able to do many of the projects around his property that used to give him a sense of purpose. And although he wasn't young at 65, neither was he an old man, and the thought of continuing to lose his mobility due to his ailments frightened him.

Joe specifically mentioned that he was an "action kind of guy" and he wanted to learn some tools that he could actively use, instead of listening passively to a hypnosis recording. While many of Kelley's clients look forward to and enjoy kicking back with a recording, she understood that Joe had a great need to take an active role in his healing. She also knew that laughter therapy was the answer.

Kelley proceeded to explain to Joe the benefits of simply laughing unconditionally – how engaging in laughter, even without humorous external stimuli, triggers the release of endorphins and increases oxygen flow, reducing suffering from pain. She also described how laughing provides a healthy massage to the internal organs, improving energy flow and vitality which was crucial for someone with Crohn's

Disease.

Joe agreed to give it a try and they started out with one of Kelley's favorite laughter recipes:

Laugh Away the Pain

It's estimated that well over 100 million Americans suffer from chronic pain, including approximately 47% of adults who experience back or neck, leg or knee, or other types of ongoing, persistent pain. Chronic pain is usually defined as pain that persists for more than three months, even occurring after injuries or surgeries have healed.

Chronic pain can drain a person of happiness and vitality. We work with pain clients in our hypnosis practices and know that there are many ways to reduce the suffering. Sometimes, a client has been trying hard to ignore the pain, having been told by their doctor that they will just have to live with it. This strategy can work, especially if the person if busy and has lots of distractions.

More often, the pain signal, instead of going away, just gets louder until the person is exhausted from all of the energy it takes to try not to listen. Here's our approach for staying ahead of pain:

Begin by focusing on the area of your body that is hurting. For the sake of this explanation, let's say there is degenerative joint pain in your knees. You can sit quietly and bring all of your attention to your knees and notice what sensations you find. You might even imagine that your knees are talking to you; what are they saying? Feel free to answer them, if you like.

You can calibrate the feelings you experience, perhaps using a mental pain scale or you may prefer to use the HOPE Coaching Comfort Scale that Kelley co-developed with Michael Ellner, because it really is more comfortable than the traditional pain scale! In fact, we suggest that you think about using that four-letter word, *pain*, less and less and replace it with *discomfort* and even better, *COMFORT*.

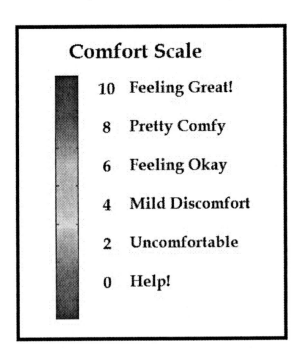

Comfort Scale

10 **Feeling Great!**

8 **Pretty Comfy**

6 **Feeling Okay**

4 **Mild Discomfort**

2 **Uncomfortable**

0 **Help!**

Next, think about the pace of that pain. That might sound rather strange but when you close your eyes, you can imagine a motion to it... even a speed to the motion. It's common that the more intense the pain signal is, the *faster* its pace.

Notice also the tone of that pain. If you were to hear it on a scale, what would the pitch of it be?

So, with the speed of your sensations in your mind, begin to laugh out loud, matching that speed and pitch with your laugh. Chances are that you sound a little bit kooky, but don't worry because you will soon be feeling better.

Keeping with the laughter, begin to slow the pace down and lower the pitch. Let this happen gradually, over a minute or so. I wonder when you will notice that your pain level is dropping (or your comfort level is rising) accordingly?

You can laugh away your pain whenever you wish. Maybe you only need to change it a bit in order to win the day or maybe you need to find big relief so that you can get a good night's rest. You get to choose! Have fun with it and make it your own natural, always with you remedy for pain!

TIP: It's important that you discern when a pain signal needs to be responded to. It would not be advisable to use any of our strategies for ignoring pain that should receive medical attention or that is serving a beneficial purpose, such as limiting unhelpful physical activities.

PS ~ Kelley's client, Joe, loved this approach and he started using it daily to stay ahead of his chronic pain. He took great pleasure in surprising his grown children with his sudden laughing outbursts, which brought them closer as a family as they saw the lighter side of their father. Within a couple of weeks Joe was stepping back into his life with a happier, more energized perspective.

Tap-n-Laugh for Pain Relief

Many people are familiar with various forms of energy psychology approaches, modalities that consider and employ the mental, emotional and physical aspects toward healing. Examples of these are acupuncture, acupressure and Reiki. Practitioners of these arts/sciences subscribe to the belief that all of our life experiences are "downloaded" into not just our brains, but into our bodies.

These approaches also involve the idea that we are all, at a quantum level, energy and that we are constantly exchanging, depleting and renewing our energy fields.

In the 1980's, Dr. Roger Callahan helped a patient by tapping underneath her eye. A student of his, Gary Craig further developed a process based on combining thoughts and feelings with stimulating the designated energy meridians of the body.

Current research demonstrates the efficacy of Craig's process in helping to down-regulate hyper-arousal of the limbic system, releasing serotonin in the amygdala, which has been described as the "smoke detector" of the body.

This tapping practice has become quite well known and is commonly called EFT (Emotional Freedom Techniques). Many hypnosis practitioners incorporate EFT and its spin-offs into their work and there is a long-standing debate over whether EFT is actually, in itself, hypnosis.

Regardless of that, EFT can be highly effective for changing how a person feels. It has even been approved for use with veterans by the Department of Defense!

For further information about EFT, please check our Resources Section at the back of this book.

Kelley has created a variation of EFT that incorporates laughter therapy. While EFT employs focusing on certain thoughts, our Tap-n-Laugh involves tapping the energy meridian sites in time with your laugh; you set the pace and tone that feels right to you.

It's easy and fun to do and it works quickly. Here's how:

Note: if tapping is uncomfortable for you, due to head or facial infirmities, you can instead gently rub in a circular motion.

It is helpful to assess how you feel before and after doing a set of EFT, so close your eyes and measure your comfort level. You can use a scale of 1-10, wherein 1 is less comfortable and 10 is more or, you can let 1 be total comfort and 10 be a high level of discomfort – you get to choose.

Next, start to gently tap with your dominant hand's index and middle fingers onto your other hand's "karate chop" point (see diagram on below).

As you do, laugh lightly out loud. Tap and laugh 10-20 times.

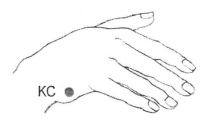

KC

Now, using the same tapping fingers, tap on the points indicated in the diagram below, starting at the top of your head and moving down. Tap 8-10 times on each point, laughing as you do.

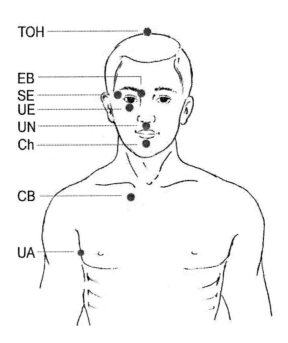

Once you finish the tapping sequence, stop and measure your current level of comfort. If it is not yet ideal, repeat the course. You will notice that with each subsequent series of tapping and laughing, you feel better and better!

The great thing about EFT and laughter is that you can do it anywhere, anytime. Have fun with it and notice that very quickly, both emotional and physical states start to become self-regulated!

Laugh and Pace Away Pain

This exercise utilizes a recipe from HOPE Coaching that Kelley created following some difficulty she had with foot pain during a karate workout. She accidentally discovered that engaging her creative imagination by "seeing" and walking a number pattern on the floor helped her quickly reduce her pain levels.

You can start by calibrating the level of your discomfort (or comfort, if you prefer our Comfort Scale).

Next, pick an area of the floor that is about four or five feet square and has no obstacles. Visualize a giant number "9" on the floor, paying attention to your breath. Take a nice deep, comfortable breath...release it and begin to walk the number, starting at the center of it. You can take small steps, you can place your feet heel-to-toe, whatever feels right for you.

With each step that you take, laugh out loud. You can laugh softly, if that feels right to you or you can let out a loud, whoop of a laugh. As always, the choice is yours.

As you near the "tail" of the "9", imagine that it loops back and leads into an "8". Keep your laughing pace and circle through the loops of the "8", enjoying the sensation of curving and breathing freely as you do so.

The "8" leads you to the top of a "7", which brings you down into a "6"...and you are already feeling better. You are probably even smiling as you laugh and experience this fun pacing exercise.

Let your feet walk along the numbers as they continue reducing... "5", "4", "3"...and does the "2" remind you of a swan? Drifting easily there, gliding gently along? You may even want to pace a couple of "2"s – because swans like to be in pairs, don't they? (Has your laughter changed to reflect your increase in comfort?)

Eventually you can cease your pacing, when you are ready to notice that you are feeling so much better. If you'd like to measure your level of comfort, go ahead. You can walk away from your pain, now...stepping out straight and strong along that line of the "1"...ready to enjoy your day. Let out one, victorious laugh to celebrate feeling better!

If you are able to, and it's convenient, laugh and pace outdoors! Connecting with Mother Nature is wonderful and when we walk barefoot on earth or grass, or maybe some soft moss, we absorb all of her beneficial properties of healing.

Not able to walk?! Not a problem: your creative imagination doesn't differentiate between real and fantasy. Take it for a spin, laughing and pacing in your mind to a better place!

Dial Up Your Comfort

In Chapter Four, *Laughter Recipes*, we shared one technique that allows you to "dial up" your Giggle Factor. Using imagery of control mechanisms, such as dials, levers, switches, etc., is an effective hypnosis approach for pain relief.

Use the Dial method, adding some other controls for yourself. For example, while you are giggling, you might imagine that you are dialing down discomfort and dialing up comfort. If a certain temperature provides you with relief, adjust that in the same way, pacing it with your laughter.

Can you laugh "up" relaxation while laughing "down" tension? (We know that typically tension contributes to pain.)

Don't forget to include mastery over the perceptions, understandings and meanings that you apply to your pain experience. If you are sick and tired of feeling depressed about having chronic pain, you have the ability to lighten those heavy feelings: dial them down with every chuckle.

Tap into your controls for feeling hopeful, loved and even joyful. Laugh up helpful and healing feelings while turning down and even muting those that are not helpful and healing.

Chapter Nine   Laughter for Self-Regulation

"Laughter gives us distance. It allows us to step back from an event, deal with it and then move on."

~ Bob Newhart

Pattern Interrupt

Neuro Linguistic Programming (NLP) is a field closely related to hypnosis. In fact, NLP is often described as conversational hypnosis. Another common way to describe NLP is "the study of the structure of subjective experience." By exploring how a person's mind organizes memories and sensory inputs, expresses metaphors, and feels emotionally about various thoughts, we can often understand how they create and perpetuate their behaviors, beliefs, and sometimes even unconsciously manifest physical symptoms.

The field of NLP emerged in the 1970's by studying and modeling the techniques of the most successful therapists of the time. One of these people was Dr. Milton H. Erickson, a psychiatrist renowned for his innovative use of hypnosis. Another was a marriage and family therapist named Virginia Satir. One of Satir's most influential insights was that the strongest human drive is toward the familiar. As a result, NLP frequently helps us identify patterns - both those responsible for undesired outcomes as well as those that generate top levels of excellence.

As hypnotists and NLP practitioners, our role then is often to interrupt unhelpful patterns that the subconscious causes to automatically repeat. Think back to the value based exercises described in Chapter Four. The idea there was that laughter can become a new and more useful response pattern compared to the more familiar stress, anxiety, anger, etc. Practicing those laughter exercises, therefore, can help you learn to interrupt your own patterns.

For the practitioner, when you've built enough rapport with a client you can afford to "spend" some of it by directly interrupting patterns in real time using some of the other techniques we've mentioned. Gibberish is one example. If you start talking nonsensically when you first meet someone it may be difficult to build trust and respect. But when you are deeply connected with someone whom you observe slipping into one of their unhelpful patterns (say, the tendency to describe a problem when being asked about the desired outcome), responding with Gibberish can interject levity, silliness and even confusion that opens a window to trance - or more likely interrupts the familiar "problem trance" the client is demonstrating.

Dave recognizes this as a familiar dynamic from the dinner table of his youth. Dad would come home from a long day at the office and in a very serious manner tell Mom all about his work day during supper. To interrupt Dad's pattern Dave would frequently interject non sequiturs that could be counted on to make Mom laugh and make it difficult for Dad to maintain his demeanor.

Anchoring Laughter

Neurons that fire together, wire together. This is neurology 101 and explains why repeated exposure to a particular stimulus will produce a consistent response. The stimulus/response relationship is called an anchor.

Anchors can be thought of as triggers for automatic patterned responses. As we go about our lives, such triggers occur all the time. Each of our sensory systems (sight, sound, smell, taste, and touch) is capable of and indeed likely to be involved in such stimulus/response pairs.

Perhaps there is a smell that reminds you of your grandma's kitchen or a song that reminds you of a past lover.

Surely this image requires no text for you to recognize its common meaning, especially if you imagine that it is colored red:

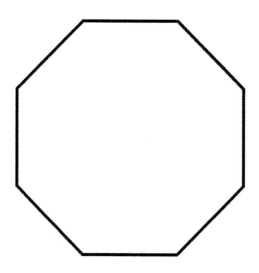

Clearly, anchors develop naturally throughout our lives. They can also be created on purpose. The classic example is Pavlov's dogs - the Russian scientist trained dogs to salivate at the sound of a tuning fork by pairing the sound with exposure to meat, noticing first that the food was a natural anchor for this physiological response and that the pairing lead to a "conditioned" response prompting salivation when the meat was ultimately removed from the equation.

In NLP and hypnosis we often help clients install anchors as shortcuts to accessing their inner resources, including laughter. Even while conducting public laughter yoga classes, Dave encourages participants to notice when they're feeling that delightful strain in their jaw or cheeks, and to set an anchor for that feeling by touching two finger tips together.

You can start developing this anchor for yourself now by consistently touching the same two finger tips together each time you laugh. Before long you'll be able to just touch those finger tips together and either notice happy feelings, find yourself laughing, or both!

Mindful Laughter

As hypnosis practitioners, we often operate via a level of *mindful hypnosis* – a practice that involves an active and participating part of the mind, rather than one that is shut down and "asleep." As mentioned earlier, that's why we may even refer to ourselves as *de*-hypnotists, helping people to wake up to the amazing abilities of their mind/body when it comes to healing and generally living in better ways.

Mindfulness is steeped in Eastern traditions of meditation

and refers to the value of being in the moment as opposed to being stuck in unhelpful timeline states. Examples of those states might be when a person is ruminating about the past or when a person is worrying about the future. It's usually more beneficial and enjoyable to be in the moment, enjoying the here and now.

Laughter therapy lends itself beautifully to the practice of mindfulness, particularly due to its premise of laughing unconditionally with the expectation of good feelings and health benefits. Releasing judgment and just allowing yourself to laugh is incredibly freeing!

Teaching a client to laugh in this way is an awesome experience. It can be done in a full waking state, of course, understanding that the mere engagement of laughing immediately begins to move us into a place that is more helpful and healing.

Combining laughter exercises with mindfulness, through awareness of breath and the physical sensations that are elicited is an easy recipe. Kelley asks a client, *"When do you think you might laugh like this?"* to ignite a mental rehearsal on their behalf. We encourage people to laugh regularly, several times a day, to help their physiology begin to self regulate.

Emotional Detox Laughter

One of our favorite HOPE Coaching techniques to help people move out of unhelpful states such as stress, anxiety, emotional and even physical discomfort, is called an anchor collapse. This too relies on the basics of neurology, allowing us to intentionally choose a new, more desirable anchored response to extinguish or neutralize another less useful anchor that likely developed naturally and perpetuated as Satir observed, simply because it had become familiar.

Once learned, this is a quick and easy mechanism that affords a person control over how they are thinking and feeling. We like that.

Kelley decided to merge the benefits of laughter therapy with the anchor collapse process called Emotional Detox and came up with a powerful and fun version. Here it is:

> Begin by allowing yourself awareness of whatever is bothering you. You may notice within your internal dialogue, distressing words, phrases, ideas, images or emotions, or you may notice it in the way your body is reacting. It's interesting that our body is always responding to whatever we are experiencing, whether we are aware of it or not. Notice that you don't even have to define what exactly it is that is taking away from your peace and comfort; you just know that it's happening.

> Once you have that awareness, go ahead and measure your reaction. You can use a scale of 1-10 where 1 is little response and 10 is a really big one. Calibrate your current level.

> Next, make a fist of your right hand and as you do, laugh out loud. Make it a strong, extended, "Ha, Ha, Ha!" Then, open your hand.

> Take a nice, deep breath and gently close and open your eyes.

Now, imagine yourself enjoying a perfect day for you. You are doing something that you really love. Maybe you are there with others or maybe you are there by yourself. Wherever you are, you feel great! It's a perfect hair day, you are healthy and comfortable and you have a big smile on your face. As you are experiencing all of the positive elements of this, make a fist with your left hand and laugh as you do, this time with a strong, extended, "Ho, Ho, Ho". Then open your hand.

Take a nice, deep breath and gently close and open your eyes.

Take a few moments to let your thoughts clear. You might imagine them as being like leaves, gently drifting down into a slowing moving stream of water, gliding away to wherever thoughts go when we don't need them anymore.

Now, here's where the magic happens: Take both hands, place them into fists and laugh out loud 5 times, "Hee, Hee, Hee, Hee, Hee!" Open and relax your hands.

Enjoy another comfortable deep breath and the relaxed feeling that you now have. Feels good, doesn't it? You can notice that original distressful thought or feeling has really decreased and it may even have totally dissipated!

You will find that with repeated application, old, stuck and useless feelings begin to permanently fade away, leaving room for positive helpful and healing ones. Use this to not only gain power over your life experience but to *stay ahead* of unnecessary stress, anxiety or other discomfort.

(Credit to Michael Ellner, Richard Jamison and Alan Barsky for the original Emotional Detox recipe)

Bilateral Stimulation Laughter

We often teach our hypnosis clients bilateral stimulation as an effective tool for reducing anxiety. Based on the scientific theory that when a person is stuck in anxious states, one hemisphere of their brain is overactive, doing a simple exercise helps bring the brain back into balance.

Here's how:

Select an object to hold. Something like a hand ball, an apple, even a pen or a set of keys will suffice. Hold the object out directly in front of you in one hand, focusing your eyes upon it.

Now begin to move the item out to one side, then back to center where you exchange it to the other hand. Continue moving it out to the other side, then back, exchanging it once again.

As you do this back and forth exchange, keep your eyes focused on the object. Don't move your head back and forth; just your eyes, following your hand movement.

We suggest that you time the passing back and forth action to the same pace of your anxious feeling. It's interesting how anxiety has a pace, isn't it? Usually quick, and often fast.

So, you've got your hands moving the object back and forth quickly and your eyes are following along. Now, add some laughs. Each time you exchange the item to a different hand, exhale a nice, loud, "Ha!" and each time that you extend the item out to the side, before returning it back to center, exhale a nice, loud, "Ha!"

You'll find that you begin to put a bit of a rhythmic and even musical pattern to the movement. Now comes the magical part:

Begin to slow down your hand movement, keeping the laughs in sync. Slow it down with each and every pass of the object and watch what happens. Within a very brief amount of time, your anxiety levels also slow and drop, your mind/body is calibrating along to your command – how cool is that?!

After only a minute or two of laughing with bilateral stimulation, you notice that you have slowed all of that anxiety down and you feel calm, at peace. What we really like about this technique is that you don't have to think about anything...you can just use the exercise for no other reason than for the health of it!

It's so easy and can be done practically anywhere. In fact, you don't even need to have an object to hold; you can imagine holding and passing something from hand to hand, clapping them together as you do so.

No Pee-Pee Hee-Hee

Kelley found that many of her female clients were stifling their natural inclinations to laugh and when she asked why, she got the answer, *"I don't want to pee my pants!"* What a shame that a physical issue prevents people from enjoying the healing benefits of laughter. In an effort to turn that around, Kelley started to encourage these clients to do some Bladder Laughter Training. Along with the kegel exercises and urine flow control described below, she had them add some gentle laughter. Simultaneous use of two different sets of muscles, pelvic and diaphragm, aids in developing better urine control.

One of the traditional contra-indications for laughter therapy is incontinence – loss of urinary control. The reason for this is that in some cases, when done improperly by contracting the abdominal muscles, laughter can actually heighten the problem. Learning how to laugh correctly can make all the difference when it comes to improving bladder control.

There are two primary classes of incontinence – one, stress incontinence, occurs at times of laughing or other experiences that put pressure on the bladder. Women who have given birth are vulnerable to this type of bladder leakage due to stretched muscles. Specific physical exercises can help the muscles regain their strength and losing excess weight will relieve pressure on internal organs and the bladder.

The other type of incontinence is urge incontinence, also known as overactive bladder. This can occur from problems such as a temporary bladder infection or chronic issues such as multiple sclerosis, diabetes, stroke or other disease. Irritation of the bladder may be a cause, so taking a nutritional approach is an option for urge incontinence.

Although there are medications that can help with incontinence, lifestyle changes are a great way to reduce and minimize episodes of urinary leakage. One of the easiest remedies is to practice pelvic wall strengthening exercises. Here are two simple exercises that are useful to men and women (locate the pelvic wall muscles by simulating trying to hold in a fart!):

1. *Kegel Laugh*

- Start with lying on your back, which makes it easier to isolate the muscles.
- Keep the muscles in your buttocks, legs and abdomen as relaxed as possible and don't hold your breath.
- Contract your pelvic muscles for a count of five and then release to a count of five.

With each "squeeze" of the pelvic muscles, laugh from the diaphragm, as described earlier in our book. It can be just a mild chuckle, that's fine. As you begin to get in touch with your body, you will recognize just the level of effort that is comfortable and right for you. If you feel any strain or urge, back off to a milder laugh. The goal is to strengthen your muscles, so building up gradually is the way to go.

2. *Stop and Go Flow*

- Halfway through urination, try to stop or slow down the flow of urine.

When urinating, practice stopping and starting the flow of urine. This action will strengthen the muscles involved in urinary control. When you are able to do this easily, add a laugh or two. Now, perhaps people will really wonder what the joke is when they hear laughter emanating from the toilet stall, but who cares?! Imagine being free of that annoying leak problem and what a relief that is...

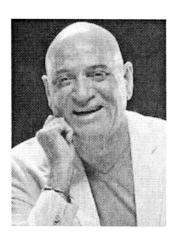

An Interview with Dr. Madan Kataria, Founder of Laughter Yoga Movement

In preparation for writing this book, Dave reached out to the founder of laughter yoga, Dr. Madan Kataria, and was delighted to not only hear back from him but be granted an online interview with this fascinating man from India. Things only got better when Dr. Kataria agreed to write the foreword for this book and we are very grateful for his time in helping us share the wonderful possibilities of laughter therapy.

Here are the highlights from Dave's interview with Dr. Kataria:

(We love how Dave's interview with Dr. Kataria started and we wish you could hear the LAUGHTER!)

D: Dr. Kataria, thank you for doing this interview. It is for a book about the health benefits of laughter, and especially how it fits with my work as a clinical and medical hypnotist. One of the reasons that I am so excited about this is I see a connection between laughter and hypnosis. They work on the same premise. In hypnosis, we say the body can't tell the difference between what is real and what is vividly imagined. In laughter yoga we say the body can't tell the difference between real laughter and enthusiastic self-simulated or fake laughter. Your brain is going to do the same thing and your body is going to get the same benefits. It is this common mechanism that got me interested in combining the two.

Dr. K: Yes, right. Hypnosis and laughter yoga concept has similarity: doing something and thinking about doing something; not much difference.

D: Tell me about your medical career? What kind of doctor are you? What kind of patients were you seeing and what kind of issues were you helping people with?

Dr. K: To bring more validation to the concept of laughter yoga I will even go before medical career, right from my childhood days...where I was born and how it came to be: I was born in a small village and we were eight brothers and sisters. And nobody was interested in education so we are into farming. When I was a child we lived in a very small village, population: 250.

People lived very naturally, we laughed a lot and surprisingly, I never heard anyone telling jokes in the village, in my entire childhood. Nobody knew what is a joke, what is a comedy, what is a sense of humor– nobody understands in villages. But still we laughed a lot. How we laughed when we were kids:

1. being together with family, something happens and we laugh

2. India is a culture where people celebrate festivals (singing, dancing, prayers, laughing). I noticed that in festivals as a kid, we laughed and laughed and laughed and still I noticed

it wasn't because there was anything funny. Being together was part of joy and laughter.

3. whenever we are at any marriage functions, social gatherings...all the time we are laughing.

My mother dreamed that one of her sons should become a doctor, because there was no medical facility in the village. So she inspired me to become a doctor, because I was good in studies. The village had a primary school and my teacher told my mother that her son was brilliant and said, "Why don't you send him to the city and get him educated?" So my mother started saying I should become a doctor. I followed my mother's dream, studied and became a medical doctor.

When I moved to city life from village, I found that all the time in the cities, people stop others from laughing, rather than encouraging people to laugh. "Stop yourself. What's so funny? Behave yourself in the name of discipline and sophistication and looking good."

So people are all the time sacrificing and not laughing much. Even the natural instinct - when we were in the village everyone was natural, burping, farting, but when we fart in the city, everyone goes, "Ah, ah, ah." *(Dr. K and Dave both laugh)*

Then it seems that it was the city life that becomes more restrictive; this is how I noticed and the same thing happens with laughing. If somebody laughs loudly, everybody is looking at this person, "Why are you laughing? What's so funny?"

And then I started to hear, when I became a doctor, about sense of humor, jokes, etc. I didn't really identify with jokes but I had a natural ability to laugh whenever we were together with people. I became a general physician in 1978, and then I came to Bombay [now called Mumbai] for post grad work to become a cardiologist.

I cleared Part I and something happened that made me lose my inspiration for medical career due to many reasons – one is that medical practice is too commercialized, pharmacy reps with gifts asking me to sell their medications and promote brands, in Bombay there was a funny thing like kickbacks...that really hurt me, I didn't like that. So even though I got money from somebody as a referral fee, I was feeling guilty about keeping it so I didn't give it back but I gave it away to the poor people.

This is where I found, and also as a physician, the best thing about allopathy, modern medicine, was surgery. Surgery has fantastic results. Intensive care unit, there is no substitute. You have to save your life, you have to go to ICU otherwise you can't rely on conventional treatments. But in day to day life I found too much of medication being prescribed even for common ailments. Too much use of antibiotics, too much use of pain killers.

And also I realized that 70% of illness is stress related, a lot of psychosomatic things are coming up. Even organic diseases, like for example chronic lung diseases - we found that 50% element is organic disease and 50% is still a mental reaction to disease. So more and more diseases of unknown etiology, we know the cause but we don't know the treatment. Allergic disorders, can't do anything. Ideopathic diseases, can't do anything.

I thought there has to be some way to integrate different systems of healing. We cannot replace modern medicine, this is a fact I acknowledge, but modern medicine does not answer all the questions. So people cannot afford modern medicine, it is becoming too expensive beyond the reach of people, especially in India. There are too many poor people in India.

Then I thought that the best way would be to integrate different systems of healing so that we can cut down on the needs of allopathic medicines. For example, if we could use homeopathy, acupuncture so that we can reduce the need for pain killers.

So I started a magazine called, *My Doctor,* to educate common man about which system to follow for which kind of diseases. We can't cure everything with allopathy but there are some things we can do to reduce suffering of symptoms with other medicines. I found miracle things in homeopathy. I found that if you follow some naturopathic principles, yoga...in that quest, my magazine I used to have different doctors from different systems of healing as panelists. I used to study, write articles on different systems...my approach towards medicine was about integrating different systems of healing.

D: Did that ever include hypnosis?

Dr. K: Yes, I read about hypnosis. I tried a few articles on hypnosis but there are not many people here in India doing hypnosis, but there are some.

I thought of writing an article about laughter is the best medicine, how laughter could help. After finding so many benefits in my research about laughter, I thought, "Such a good medicine, nobody laughs in Mumbai, everybody is so serious."

So the idea came to me, "Why not start a Laughter Club?!"

D: And the rest is history! So, do you still practice medicine?

Dr. K: I stopped practicing medicine in 2001.

D: How quickly did laughter yoga spread beyond the park in Mumbai where you started?

Dr. K: Quickly means within 10 days we were in the national newspapers, national television about the new idea of laughter club. I started on the 13th of March, 1995, and everybody started calling and visiting our park; journalists from all over the world, news agencies, Associated Press. There were several people from different countries. Our park was full every day with journalists.

I started getting calls from everywhere. Within one month, we established 13 laughter yoga clubs in Mumbai.

And it seemed that everybody was an expert because all the members knew this exercise, but I told them to make their own exercise. I said the best guidelines: Laugh for no reason – just fake it 'til you make it! And in between you breathe and do some stretching exercises and that's it – that's laughter yoga!

The greatest thing that happened to laughter yoga is that I never thought of making it a business or franchise. Whoever asked me to start a laughter club, I came to their park for one hour to teach and the next day they had a laughter club! It was so easy, there was no money involved in this.

So I traveled all over India for almost next 5 yrs, '95-'99. I spent all of my savings. I was missing my medical practice, so my practice was going down and that was not funny.

In 1999 I was invited to the United States, by a psychologist named Stevenson. My wife and I visited 14 cities and made over 40 presentations. It seemed that America loved this idea and it started spreading in America. Then I went to Australia, we went to Germany, and it just started spreading globally.

In about 2003/4 started a teacher training system so I didn't have to go everywhere; we created Leader Training and now we have Master Trainers so that I can sit quiet and laugh!

I think that one of the reasons for the success of laughter yoga is that I did not put laughter yoga in a box, telling them that my way is the right way. There are only these guidelines: that we laugh for no reason, no use of jokes or comedies, breathe, take long deep breaths, unconditional love, fake it 'til you make it, stretch in between and play like children.

D: Did you imagine laughter yoga would become so popular?

Dr. K: The way media as well as people all over the world got interested and started calling me, I started to feel that this is something bigger, something really big, but I didn't expect that it would be so fast. I kept working hard, developing and innovating the ideas, not only social laughter clubs but started thinking about senior centers, thinking about seniors who could not run around. So we started developing ideas for seniors.

Then we started thinking about laughter yoga for school children. Children can sing, jump, laugh and play so we made different ways for children. Then, how do physically and mentally challenged people need laughter, according to their abilities and physical limits. Then we went to prison systems; they need it the most because there is too much anger there.

We went everywhere and I realized that this is an idea that is suitable for all age groups, from childhood to old age - from womb to tomb!

D: Now that laughter yoga is so well established, what do you see in the future, going forward?

Dr. K: I think that the most focus of laughter yoga is social laughter clubs – social networking - all over the world. But I am seeing possibilities in more and more research popping up. I see business people using it as laughter yoga can resolve issues they have.

Laughter is most needed in the schools so I see that in each and every company, ten years from now, there will be a lot of in-house laughter sessions in work places, schools and colleges. We already started with one here in Bangalore. There is a laughter yoga classroom here, we go every day for a 30 minute period and there are several other places in India where we have official laughter yoga classes.

D: Wow, I'd like to go to a school like that (both men laugh).

Dr. K: Yeah, it might happen everywhere. So I'm seeing that if you want to change the world, catch them young. Children need to learn to laugh and be playful – that will help them for the rest of their life.

Additionally, there are millions of people in old age homes all over the world. Each and every old age home might have one certified laughter leader teacher in house, there will be laughter yoga classes in the senior centers.

I also see that there are millions of people in the prison system so there will be a regular laughter session there. All NGO's like for physically, mentally challenged, blind school, you name anything...so practically, I am expecting an explosion of laughter around the world!

D: (laughing and clapping) Very Good, Very Good, YAY!

Dr. K: So my role is I have to see and develop the applications of laughter yoga, create new systems, oversee some scientific research. That is why I am busy now, setting up Laughter University here in Bangalore which will be the clearing house for teaching coaching training systems around the world, so that it goes on uninterrupted, even after I leave this planet.

D: I want to ask you about specific research in this area. There are some studies that have been cited, in the area of pain and other chronic illness. I am interested in research regarding pain, automimmune disease and other chronic illness. Also, concepts of placebo and nocebo - we are talking about things like neuroplasticity, which people understand to be re-wiring the brain, but when it comes to changing how physiology in general is able to shift, we call that bioplasticity. What are you doing in the area of research?

Dr. K: I follow quite a few research studies in different countries, for example, in Germany, about laughter yoga and depression. There was already one study in Iran measuring the effect of laughter yoga on depression with elderly people. So I see that for measuring the effect of laughter on depression, which is the number one sickness in the world today, we don't need any physiological parameters. Psychometrics are good enough to measure the level of depression, the effect of depression on body and mind.

So that's the theory. Depression being so prevalent worldwide, I think this is something that is going to be a breakthrough in mental health. At the anecdotal level, I have thousands of testimonials from my students and people who have joined laughter clubs.

As far as biological research is concerned, to see the physiological changes happening in the body as a result of laughter exercises, the best thing, I would still say, is measuring the effects of stress on the body, such as cortisol level in saliva which is the biggest indication of stress, blood pressure, and heart rate variability. That's another parameter which has been used in many studies. I did use it in some research that hasn't been published...

(The online connection was breaking up a bit here...and Dr. Kataria started to laugh, saying that perhaps it was a sign

to take a break from such serious talk and just laugh!)

Dr. K: My focus now is with the business world and with children. What I tell them is let us laugh but at the same time measure the effect of laughter, mostly using psychometric testing. One of the best outcomes of laughter yoga, I feel, is developing emotional intelligence, meaning that negative emotions go down and positive emotions go up in a measurable way.

I have figured out some psychometric tests measuring the Emotional Intelligence of the employees that will help them a lot in the business world. One is called Firo B. You can Google it and see for yourself what it is.

People are always talking about Emotional Intelligence, but I don't see easy tools for developing Emotional Intelligence.

D: My take on Emotional Intelligence also has to do with having the ability to understand and perceive where other people are at, so you can be more sensitive to them.

Dr. K: Yes, understanding your own emotions and understanding other people's emotions, so you can relate with them. Also, for me, Emotional Intelligence is about self-regulation, for example how powerful you are to control your senses. Emotions will take you to the right places or emotions will take you to the wrong places. Are you going with the emotions without rationalizing them; sometimes are you able to say, "No!"

So, how do you talk to your mind? You are different than mind. This is the awareness that laughter yoga brings that you are not your mind, you are different from your mind, so that you can identify where you are going so you can stop yourself if you are going to do something that is disastrous for you, as well as for other people.

Another part of Emotional Intelligence I feel is about empathy, sensitivity to the difficulties and suffering of other people. If you develop generosity, sensitivity, that kind of giving, and we have been noticing all this in laughter yoga clubs! People are becoming very generous. People are becoming very helping. This is a big part of laughter yoga's outcome - empathy. I feel that Emotional Intelligence is not just about positive and negative emotions, this is a huge part.

So, honestly I have not found many tools for helping people become emotionally intelligent. Laughter yoga is very powerful, very simple, very effective when it comes to being with your emotions and it works much faster. The reason being is that it is a body-oriented technique; emotions at the body level involve diaphragmatic breathing and movement. The seat of emotions is your breathing, so setting your breathing right also helps you regulate your emotions in a much better way.

D: You mentioned before, the heart rate variability and recently I have been reading about the vagus nerve and specifically the vagal tone...about the difference between how long you are exhaling compared to how long you are inhaling – do you see that being connected to the importance of breathing in laughter?

Dr. K: Yes. Movement of the diaphragm actually activates the vagus nerve which is carrying parasympathetic nerve fibers. Diaphragmatic belly breathing, belly laughing helps to increase the vagal tone, the parasympathetic reaction, so that we have less stress reactions.

D: The book, Anatomy of an Illness, *by Norman Cousins, is mentioned in the same breath with laughter yoga as great examples of healing of laughter. When did you read it and what do you think of it?*

Dr. K: I read about Norman Cousins before I wrote my article, before I started my laughter club.

D: Cousins talked about the placebo effect. Can you comment about that and also about the nocebo effect, when it comes to the health benefits of laughter?

Dr. K: When I think of the placebo effect when it comes to laughter, I think there is nothing wrong with it. There are two effects: one is the effect on the mind, the other is the effect on the body.

Nobody can deny that when you are exhaling in laughter you are getting more oxygen exchange for the carbon dioxide and you are increasing your breathing capacity by the breathing exercises. But at the mental level, if someone thinks I am getting better with laughter, there is nothing wrong with it. So it's a mix of physical and psychological; I feel it's a mixture of body and mind supporting each other.

As a medical doctor, I have been seeing that 50% of the cause of illness is physical; organic disease as a cause of illness. But more than 50%, I would say, is a mental reaction to illness – what is happening, will I die?, will I be crippled? Mental reactions that are too much.

D: That's the nocebo effect.

Dr. K: Yes. So I think rather than placebo I would say that laughter yoga has a powerful effect against nocebo.

D: You are confirming a lot of what I have come to believe through my hypnosis practice. Although you said that there are not a lot of hypnotists in India, have you talked to any other hypnotists around the world who are combining laughter with hypnosis in the way we are talking about?

Dr. K: Although there are hypnotists in India, by chance I

have not met them. In other countries there are a lot of hypnotists who follow laughter yoga and they are reaffirming and confirming what we are talking about – neuroplasticity, and now the subject, bioplasticity, that you brought up and makes a lot of sense to me.

D: What would you say motivates you, keeps you so inspired to be the worldwide leader of laughter yoga?

(both men laugh)

Dr. K: First, that if I don't feel the benefits of laughter myself, I cannot be motivated. I laugh every day in the morning for 30, 40, 50 minutes all by myself. So that gives me energy in the morning so I feel full of energy for the day and is also wonderful motivation for me. This is really cool stuff, not a theory, if it is working on you. A lot of people can teach other people but they cannot experience for themselves. So this is one motivation.

The second motivation for me is when I see people getting so many benefits; that's my motivation, getting so many messages from people all over the world, telling me how great is laughter yoga, how it has changed their lives. That's my motivation.

To be able to be useful to the world....and so quick – you don't have to wait for weeks and months; the effects, the results are almost instantaneous.

I feel that coming to laughter yoga, I found my real purpose in life. Before laughter yoga, I was pursuing some goals to achieve something great in my life that was all for myself. So after being in laughter yoga I found that the real laughter, there is nothing to achieve in this world, one has to contribute something before we leave this world, so I feel that I have done this. I have contributed something that is changing the world.

D: That is so well said, thank you. (both men laugh) Do you have any tips for laughter leaders, for leading groups?

Dr. K: I think for leaders: laughter yoga is not meant to be making a business out of it. Let business be the outcome of your good work, so you start spreading laughter to as many people as possible and money will come out of it.

D: Is there anything else you want to add?

Dr. K: I just want to bring reference to Charles Darwin and to psychologist William James, who hypothesized that bodily expression of any emotion reinforces that emotion in the mind. It is not so easy to work on the mind; it is easier to work on the body. Laughter yoga is mind/body medicine.

My own feeling is that laughter yoga would be incomplete without the yoga element.

Yoga is more than breathing, it is more about spirituality. I think laughing unconditionally brings in lots of spiritual wisdom, without knowing you have it. Like, for example, you connect with people, it changes you, makes you become much more generous. Spiritual qualities and virtues are developed with laughter yoga.

I think that without spiritual element we cannot have Emotional Intelligence because in spirituality, there are not too many hows and whys. We know from spiritual knowledge that there are certain rules of nature that you cannot question. You have to follow those rules. Spirituality can be experienced, but cannot be explained logically.

What we are trying to build, the next part, is inner spirit of laughter. If you want to get the positive effects of laughter much more quickly, we have to be aware of the spiritual wisdom to be combined that essentially comes from yoga.

116

Like for example, there are certain rules of life, spiritual laws which govern the body. For example:

Laugh impermanence. We are actually creating those exercises in laughter yoga that nothing is permanent in this world, everything is changing. Nothing is going to stay forever. So I was thinking to disseminate that knowledge, spiritual wisdom and making some laughter exercises out of it.

Laugh imperfection. Nothing is perfect. All imperfections put together become perfect. You don't have to be afraid of making mistakes, doing something wrong. If you don't do wrong, you cannot do right. You will never even get started if you think you are not perfect.

Laugh Oneness. Everything in this world belongs to you; you belong to everything. It is not a question of one person, one nation. The whole world is one community. What I'm doing is, I'm making all these laughter exercises to give these messages of spiritual wisdom, where we can understand these spiritual principles, like...

Laugh Karma. Nothing changes if you don't do it. I mean, an idea is good but you have to walk on the idea, you have to act on the idea. All these things are very, very important to live a meaningful, purposeful life.

Everything that happens in your life, there is a reason for it. So you don't have to feel guilty about it, something wrong or my bad. My destiny is not good or bad, everything is fantastic. Nature has a way to teach us to accept it, to move on, not get stuck with it. Kindness, forgiveness, all these things have to become part of life. Only then can we call it yoga.

D: I was taught that the mission of laughter yoga is to spread world peace through laughter. This seems like the natural extension of all that you just talked about.

Dr. K: Yes, health, happiness, world peace through laughter. This is our mission!

(both men laugh)

D: I am so grateful to you for the opportunity to talk with you one on one, and for the impact that your life's work has had on me and all the people in my life. Thank you!

What a wonderful way to end our book, with Dr. Kataria's wish for health, happiness and peace throughout the world through laughter.

We hope you have found not only valuable information here, but inspiration to laugh often, knowing that what you are doing is not only benefiting yourself, but others.

Feel free to contact Dave or Kelley through their website information listed. Thank you for being part of our journey!

Resources

Kelley's site – www.woodshypnosis.com

Dave's site – www.manifestpositivity.com

Dr. Kataria's site - www.laughteryoga.org

Celeste Greene's site - www.laughteryogaatlanta.com

Skype laughter club - www.facebook.com/skypelaughterclub

Laughter by phone - www.laughteryogaonthephone.com
(701) 432-3900, Code: 6071292#

Emotional Freedom Technique -
www.emofree.com, www.eftuniverse.com

HOPE Coaching - www.mindfulhypnosiscoach.com

Support this book - www.laughterforthehealthofit.com

Acknowledgements

Dave thanks Dr. Madan Kataria for his inspiration and vision; Kathleen Krauss for her years of friendship and mentorship; Celeste Greene for her friendly welcome to Atlanta; Michael Coleman for his friendly welcome to San Diego; James Hazlerig for countless conversations exploring the connections between laughter yoga and hypnotherapy; Scott Sandland and Richard Clark for opening HypnoThoughts Live to the presentation of this topic; Jane Allen for the introduction to laughter yoga; and April Martin and the staff of Om Shala Yoga in Arcata, CA for graciously providing free space to the Humboldt Laughter Club.

Kelley thanks her mother, who imbued her with an irrepressible positive mindset, her kids who keep her young and the many clients who keep teaching her the value of living life to the fullest.

About the Authors

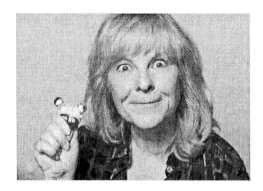

Kelley T. Woods loves to laugh, especially unconditionally. She operates a private hypnosis practice in Mount Vernon, WA, helping people of all ages improve their lives. She is the author of several books and active in the hypnosis community as both a teacher and lifelong student. www.woodshypnosis.com

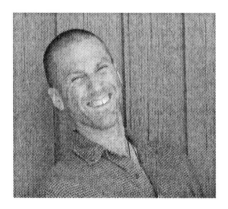

Dave Berman takes laughter very seriously. Whether leading laughter groups, working with hypnosis and coaching clients, or writing articles and books, Dave is a passionate educator about the mind/body connection and an ambassador for the laughter yoga movement. www.ManifestPositivity.com